Author's Note on the Cover Image

The bowl on the cover of this book represents kintsugi, the Japanese art of repairing broken pottery with lacquer dusted with gold. As a philosophy, kintsugi embraces the cracks in an object as part of its history that should be highlighted, not hidden.

To me, this means there is a beauty in our flaws, our grief, our experiences, good and bad. We are not broken by our tragedy, our loss, our miscarriages, but made stronger by what we learn from them.

Embrace the cracks. You are not broken.

Not Broken: An Approachable Guide to Miscarriage and Recurrent Pregnancy Loss, Second Edition

ISBN: 978-0-9987146-7-7

No part of this book may be reproduced or distributed in any way without permission from the author. The information in this book, including references, is for educational purposes only and is not intended to diagnose, treat, or cure any health problem or disease, nor is it intended to substitute for the advice of your healthcare professional. Consult your healthcare provider before taking any herbs, medications, or supplements, especially if you are pregnant or breastfeeding. Any attempt to diagnose or treat an illness should be done under the direction of your healthcare provider. The author is not responsible for any adverse effects or consequences resulting from the use of any of the suggestions provided in this book.

Copyright © 2022 Dr. Lora Shahine LLC. All Rights Reserved.

Contents

Forward	by Dr. Ruth Lathi and Rachel McGrath	7
Introduction	by Dr. Lora Shahine	9
Chapter 1	The Importance of Language: The Words We Use to Define Miscarriage and Why They Matter	12
Chapter 2	Why Me? Evaluation and Treatment of Recurrent Pregnancy Loss	23
	Chapter 2.1: Anatomic Issues, Tests, and Treatment	26
	Chapter 2.2: Genetic Issues, Tests, and Treatment	34
	Chapter 2.3: Immune Issues, Tests, and Treatment	38
	Chapter 2.4: Hormonal Issues, Tests, and Treatment	43
	Chapter 2.5: Unexplained RPL	53
Chapter 3	When Experts Disagree: Controversies in Care for Recurrent Pregnancy Loss	56
	Chapter 3.1: Blood Clotting – Testing and Treatment Controversies	59
	Chapter 3.2: Hormonal Issues – Testing and Treatment Controversies	65
	Chapter 3.3: Infection – Testing and Treatment Controversies	76
	Chapter 3.4: Immune Issues – Testing Controversies	79
	Chapter 3.5: Immune Issues – Treatment Controversies	85
	Chapter 3.6: Genetic Testing of Miscarriages	91
	Chapter 3.7: Ovarian Reserve Testing	94
	Chapter 3.8: IVF for RPL	94

Chapter 4	Genetics: The Link Between Age, Egg Quality, and Miscarriage	96
Chapter 5	Lifestyle Modifications: Optimize Health and Decrease Miscarriage Risk	113
	Chapter 5.1: Lifestyle Modifications	114
	Chapter 5.2: Environmental Exposures and Miscarriage	121
	Chapter 5.3: Practice Self-Care	127
Chapter 6	Emotional Wellness: The Psychological Impact of Miscarriage	131
Chapter 7	The Other Half: What About Men and Miscarriage?	139
Chapter 8	Planting the Seeds of Pregnancy: An Integrative Approach to Miscarriage	150
	Chapter 8.1: Introduction to Traditional Chinese Medicine	151
	Chapter 8.2: Nutrition Recommendations	155
	Chapter 8.3: Supplement Recommendations	159
	Chapter 8.4: Lifestyle Modification Recommendations	162
	Chapter 8.5: Acupuncture: Tips on What to Expect	163
Chapter 9	Now What? Moving Forward as an Advocate for Your Care	167

Glossary of Terms and Acronyms	175
References	182
About the Author	201
More Educational Resources	203
Acknowledgements	204

Forward

The first edition of *Not Broken* has been a wonderful resource for my patients dealing with miscarriage, and this second edition adds even more insight and updates in this rapidly developing area of medicine.

Dr. Shahine reviews definitions, testing, and treatment options for miscarriage from an evidence-based, Western medicine approach but also includes insight into many controversies in care. I appreciate her approach to writing: a clear and concise review of what we know and a lot of what we do not yet know about miscarriage but written in a way someone without a medical degree or scientific background can understand.

My patients have shared how much they appreciate my recommendation for this book – it answers many questions they forgot to ask at the consult, helps them understand the testing we are doing, and helps them think through the options available for moving forward.

While I am happy to have mentored Lora in her early years, I now have the privilege of working side by side with her to advance the field of recurrent pregnancy loss through research, advocacy, and education. It is wonderful to have a partner in this complex field.

I recommend this book to anyone who wants to learn more about miscarriage and recurrent pregnancy loss. *Not Broken* is a truly empowering, approachable read.

– **Dr. Ruth Lathi**, associate professor of obstetrics and gynecology and reproductive endocrinology and infertility at Stanford University Medical Center and founder and director of the Center for Recurrent Pregnancy Loss at Stanford University

Dr. Lora Shahine has written a powerful book in *Not Broken*. As someone who has suffered unexplained, recurrent miscarriages in the past, this book would have been an incredibly valuable resource to me. *Not Broken* is not full of the medical jargon and generic explanations that can be found in most resources. Instead, it contains practical and helpful information to help with the understanding of why miscarriage happens, as well as potential avenues a couple can explore if they are faced with infertility issues.

Having experienced multiple losses, I was, at the time, desperate for answers. The doctors and specialists were not always helpful, often giving me generic explanations, and progress was slow on finding a diagnosis for what I was going through. I ended up scouring the internet for answers, which in turn gave me a lot of misinformation and further anxiety. In this book, Dr. Shahine expertly explains what recurrent miscarriage is, as well as its potential causes, and provides practical advice and information. She also highlights other potential factors that may need to be considered, such as emotional and lifestyle factors.

Any woman who has experienced more than one miscarriage should read this book, even if just to provide direction and support as a way forward, and perhaps some reassurance that there are many factors at play when it comes to diagnosing the cause. *Not Broken* provides hope and empowerment for women experiencing recurrent miscarriage and hopefully a way forward and perspective toward their personal situation.

– **Rachel McGrath**, award-winning author of *Finding the Rainbow* and *Embracing the Storm*

Introduction

The title of this book is inspired by my brave, resilient patients who come to me feeling broken after a miscarriage. It does not matter how many miscarriages they've had, how far along they were when they lost their pregnancies, or who they are: miscarriage shakes them to their core. By the time they see me, miscarriages have taken away the innocence of a positive pregnancy test and left them feeling self-doubt and fear that the family they dream of will never happen.

When I started counseling patients for recurrent miscarriage, I soon realized that my patients could not process and retain all the information we discussed in our visits together. I could review each test result and treatment option and answer a battery of questions, but this field is complex, and information on the internet and social media is confusing. I searched for a resource for my patients to help with questions between visits but could not find the book I wanted. In 2015, the books available on miscarriage were either outdated, extremely technical, or focused on personal stories of hope but lacking medical education. So, I wrote *Not Broken* with my own patients in mind: an evidence-based review of what we know and don't know about miscarriage written in language (I hope) that is easy to read. I didn't shy away from controversies in the field – patients often get stuck in the middle of providers who recommend different approaches, and I wanted to review the gray areas of miscarriage too.

I self-published the first edition of *Not Broken* in 2017 with help from dear friends: my editor, Lucy Elenbaas, who also edited my first book, *Planting the Seeds of Pregnancy*, which was cowritten with Stephanie Gianarelli, LAc. Stephanie contributes the chapter on an Eastern medicine approach to miscarriage care in this book. Juli Douglas, former neighbor, friend, and incredibly talented artist, helped with the cover art and images throughout the book. I called on mentors, friends, and colleagues to help me make sure that I covered topics to the best of current knowledge and understanding, and I truly appreciate the help I was given! It really does take a village to write a book.

When the first edition of *Not Broken* was published in 2017, it was current and up to date, but medicine is constantly changing, and we're always learning more about miscarriage and reproduction. Even the definition of miscarriage and recurrent pregnancy loss has changed over time. When I was in medical training, I was taught to not start an evaluation for recurrent miscarriage until someone had suffered at least three clinical miscarriages (miscarriages at least 5-6 weeks along when pregnancy could be confirmed with ultrasound or tissue diagnosis, but this excludes earlier losses). In 2013, ASRM, the American Society of Reproductive Medicine, changed their recommendation to evaluation after two clinical miscarriages. In 2020, ASRM changed it again to be much more inclusive by removing the 'clinical miscarriage' clarification of the definition. This update, in combination with the updated research and guidelines in this ever-evolving field, inspired this second edition of *Not Broken*.

This second edition is as up to date as a printed book can be, but remember while reading that there is no single expert-agreed-upon or definitive way to approach recurrent miscarriage. Science and technology are teaching us more every day, but we still have much to learn about reproduction. Miscarriage is still a gray area of medicine, with very few well-funded, large clinical trials and research studies compared to other areas of medicine like cancer and cardiovascular disease. Few providers have been trained or feel comfortable caring for patients with recurrent miscarriage. Patients often feel alone and have difficulty finding accurate information from their providers and online. As we learn more, I walk with patients through their journey to parenthood, and I hope to pass this knowledge on to you. This book may be used as a general guide, but it cannot replace visiting a miscarriage specialist since every person and situation is unique.

If you are reading this book to learn more about your own journey, I want you to finish this book feeling more knowledgeable, to let go of any shame you might feel about miscarriage, and to feel more empowered to be an advocate for yourself and your care. Try to remember along the way what I tell my own patients:

Every pregnancy is a new opportunity, and most people with miscarriages go on to have a baby. Keep reading to learn why.

– Lora Shahine, MD, FACOG

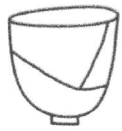

1

The Importance of Language: The Words We Use to Define Miscarriage and Why They Matter

My hope is for you to finish this book more knowledgeable about all aspects of miscarriage so you feel empowered to advocate for your care. The doctor-patient relationship is best when both participants understand, discuss, and partake during evaluation and treatment. Part of having a deeper discussion with your physician is sharing an understanding of scientific language and definitions. Clarity in language and understanding definitions of miscarriage and recurrent miscarriage are key to better understanding and communication, so we'll review them here.

Definition of Miscarriage

A miscarriage is typically defined as a pregnancy that naturally stops developing before viability. Each professional medical society has its own slight variation on the definition:

- **ASRM (American Society of Reproductive Medicine)** defines miscarriage as the naturally occurring expulsion of nonviable fetus and placenta from the uterus.[1]
- **ACOG (American Congress of Obstetricians and Gynecologists)** defines miscarriage as the loss of pregnancy at less than 20 weeks' gestation.[2]

- **ESHRE (European Society of Human Reproduction and Embryology)** defines miscarriage as pregnancy loss before viability.[3]
- **RCOG (Royal College of Obstetricians and Gynecologists)** defines miscarriage as the spontaneous loss of pregnancy before viability, the time from conception to 24 weeks' gestation.[4]

Definition of Clinical vs. Biochemical Miscarriage

Knowing the timing of a miscarriage, meaning when the pregnancy stops developing, helps doctors with evaluation and next steps in care. Your doctor may use the following terms when discussing or recording your history in your medical chart:

- **Biochemical Miscarriage** – A pregnancy that stops developing before an intrauterine pregnancy can be visualized on ultrasound or pregnancy tissue from the uterine cavity can be identified under a microscope.
- **Clinical Miscarriage** – A pregnancy that stops developing within the first trimester but after a pregnancy has been identified within the uterine cavity on ultrasound or tissue collected from the uterus is confirmed to be pregnancy tissue by histopathologic evaluation.

A pregnancy can be detected by either a urine or a blood test – both tests are designed to detect beta human chorionic gonadotropin (also known as beta HCG or bHCG), the hormone made by a pregnancy. Home urine pregnancy tests are incredibly sensitive and accurate and can detect bHCG approximately two weeks after ovulation, which is usually four weeks after the start of a period or as early as a week after ovulation in some circumstances. Someone reporting a positive home pregnancy test (urine test) followed by negative pregnancy tests and a period likely had a biochemical miscarriage. In these cases, the egg and sperm fertilized, and the resulting embryo implanted and started making bHCG, but the pregnancy stopped developing early.

Many patients have felt dismissed by doctors and loved ones while recovering from very early miscarriages. When someone is trying to build their family, a menstrual cycle is another lost month and time to grieve. Adding a positive pregnancy test followed by a late menstrual cycle may result in more loss, grief, and confusion.

We still have a lot to learn about biochemical miscarriages, causes, and treatment. We know more about clinical miscarriages with tissue that can be tested, but this does not mean we should ignore earlier biochemical miscarriages. It is important to pay attention since research shows that patients with a history of biochemical miscarriages seem to have a higher risk of more clinical miscarriages and poorer prognosis for fertility.[5,6]

Other First Trimester Issues

Miscarriages do NOT include two other pregnancy outcomes that occur in the first trimester: ectopic pregnancy and molar pregnancy.

- **Ectopic Pregnancy** – A pregnancy that develops outside of the uterine cavity, predominantly in the fallopian tubes. An ectopic pregnancy is not a viable pregnancy and must be treated (although some resolve without intervention) medically or surgically to avoid bleeding and other consequences to the pregnant woman.
- **Molar Pregnancy** – A rare pregnancy complication in which abnormal genetics in the embryo lead to irregular pregnancy growth not compatible with viability. There are different types of molar pregnancies (also called hydatidiform mole); none will result in a normal pregnancy, and all should

be treated and followed closely, because in rare instances, the tissue can grow into metastatic (cancer) disease.

Miscarriage, ectopic pregnancy, and molar pregnancy are all complications of early pregnancy but require treatment and follow up unique to each situation. Interventions like medical or surgical care help keep the patient safe. Recovery from these first trimester pregnancy complications is both physical and emotional – be sure to ask questions and care for both your physical and mental health along the way.

Definition of Recurrent Pregnancy Loss (RPL)

In 2013, ASRM defined RPL as "a disease distinct from infertility defined by 2 or more failed pregnancies."[1] They went on to state that, "for the purposes of evaluation and treatment for recurrent pregnancy loss, a pregnancy is defined as a **clinical pregnancy** documented by ultrasonography and or histopathologic examination."[1] In 2020, ASRM changed their definition of **recurrent pregnancy loss** to "a disease distinct from infertility, defined as the spontaneous loss of 2 or more pregnancies" without the limited definition of clinical pregnancy.[7] ASRM further states, "Each pregnancy loss merits careful review to determine whether specific evaluation of the woman or couple may be appropriate."[7]

Definitions and language are extremely important in developing guidelines for evaluation and treatment of any disease. Many couples have been denied testing and care for miscarriage based on previous medical definitions. Before 2013, the textbook definition of RPL required **three or more consecutive clinical miscarriages** to be documented before testing and treatment for miscarriage was recommended. In 2013, ASRM decreased the number of clinical miscarriages needed to instigate an evaluation to two and removed the 'consecutive' clause of the definition. In 2020,

ASRM removed the 'clinical pregnancy' clarification from the definition of recurrent miscarriage and opted for a more inclusive 'pregnancy,' which opens the evaluation to any pregnancy loss, regardless of gestational age. The 2020 ASRM definition clearly states that any miscarriage should be evaluated and cared for and should empower people to ask more questions and be advocates for their miscarriage care.

Medical Definitions: Why Does My Chart Say 'Abortion'?

Medical definitions of miscarriage often include the term 'abortion,' and patients can be upset reading the terms 'threatened abortion' and 'spontaneous abortion' in their medical record if they do not understand what these medical terms mean. To people outside of medicine, the term abortion is usually associated with a deliberate termination of pregnancy. However, the medical term means a premature end of a pregnancy before viability.

- **Threatened Abortion** – A pregnancy associated with bleeding or cramping but that otherwise seems viable. For example, if someone is bleeding in pregnancy, but the ultrasound is showing a fetus of the appropriate size with a heartbeat, the medical chart would classify this as a 'threatened abortion,' even though the evaluation of pregnancy is reassuring.
- **Missed Abortion** – A pregnancy that is not viable but has not been associated with common signs of miscarriage like bleeding or cramping. For example, if someone comes to a checkup visit at 10 weeks' gestation and the ultrasound shows a pregnancy measuring seven weeks in size (much smaller than expected) with no heartbeat, but there were no symptoms or warning signs that something was wrong, the medical chart would classify this as a 'missed abortion.'

The dating of a missed abortion in a medical chart can be confusing to patients. In the case discussed above, the pregnancy stopped developing at 7 weeks' gestation, but the patient had not had any signs of possible miscarriage like spotting or cramping. The miscarriage was discovered at 10 weeks' gestation at a routine prenatal ultrasound.

The medical chart will likely note both the patient's gestation (how far along they were in pregnancy) and the size of the fetus (when development stopped). This clarification is helpful for doctors so they may ask questions like this at a visit. Every miscarriage is important to evaluation – no matter how far along. If the doctor is trying to understand when your pregnancy stopped developing, it's not to dismiss it or make you feel it's less important because the miscarriage was early. They ask to help better understand how to help with testing and next steps.

- **Spontaneous Abortion** – A pregnancy that stopped developing and resolved (expelled from the uterus) without medical intervention.
- **Therapeutic Abortion** – A procedure that ends a pregnancy on purpose, either with medication or a procedure like a dilation and curettage (D&C). This term does not indicate why the pregnancy was ended (electively or for a medical reason).
- **Complete Abortion** – A pregnancy that has resolved with or without medical intervention, such as medication to help the uterus expel the pregnancy (like misoprostol) or a procedure to help empty the uterus (like a D&C).

These terms help medical providers document precisely what happened with a patient medically, but the medical use of the term "abortion" can be very confusing and even hurtful if not explained to patients who are losing a very desired pregnancy.

> I've had patients call the office in tears reading the documentation for the care for their miscarriage. The medical terms used to describe and bill for care can leave patients confused and hurt if not explained.

Scope of This Book

In this book, I will focus on first trimester miscarriages (intrauterine pregnancy losses that occur before 13 weeks' gestation). Most miscarriages occur in the first trimester, and recurrent first trimester miscarriages are the focus of my training and practice as a reproductive endocrinologist. I often consult for patients with second and third trimester pregnancy losses, but I work with a perinatologist (also known as a maternal fetal medicine specialist or a high-risk obstetrician) to help these patients. A perinatologist is an OBGYN whose training and practice focus on complicated or high-risk obstetric care later in pregnancy, such as premature labor, preeclampsia, cervical incompetence, and more. Patients with second and third trimester pregnancy losses and stillbirth will benefit from reading many aspects of this book, such as lifestyle modifications, self-care, and emotional well-being, which can improve overall physical and emotional health, but the evaluation and treatment for these later losses are outside the scope of this book.

How Common Is Miscarriage?

Miscarriage is more common than most people realize. It can occur in as many as one in four clinically recognized pregnancies.[8] The estimated incidence of miscarriage is considerably higher if earlier biochemical miscarriages are included. It's estimated that as many as 70% of fertilized eggs or embryos stop developing.

Although people are starting to talk more about miscarriage and recurrent pregnancy loss, many people still do not share their stories. Most miscarriages occur in the first trimester, before people have told friends and family or are 'showing,' and many patients are warned by their doctors to wait to share the good news 'just in case,' meaning just in case of miscarriage. I'd argue that this is when people need comfort the most, and it's tough to share the joy of pregnancy and the grief of miscarriage in the same conversation.

> When patients ask my advice on when and if to tell people they are pregnant, I suggest sharing early pregnancy with a select group of close family/friends who can be excited with you and support you if needed.

My patients are often relieved when I tell them how common miscarriages are since many of them feel isolated, like they are the only one of their family and friends who has had a miscarriage or recurrent pregnancy loss. At later visits, these same patients tell me that once they started sharing with their friends and family that they had a miscarriage, they were overwhelmed with the outpouring of support and people saying, "Oh, that happened to me too!" Miscarriage can feel isolating, but we can reduce the feelings of guilt and shame the more we share and support each other!

ASRM estimates that 15-25% of all clinically recognized pregnancies end in miscarriage, and that if biochemical miscarriages are included, the chance that a positive pregnancy test will end in miscarriage is much higher.[1]

Risk of Miscarriage and Age

The risk of miscarriage increases with advanced maternal reproductive age, as shown below in the following chart.[9]

Age in Years	Risk of Miscarriage
35-39	25%
40-44	51%
45+	93%

Patients can be shocked when I tell them that at age 40, the chance of having a baby after a positive pregnancy test is 50%. Human reproduction is extremely inefficient. One egg ovulates each cycle, but hundreds to thousands of eggs are lost in the process, regardless of whether someone is trying to conceive or is using contraception. As eggs age, fewer of them can successfully complete all the genetic requirements needed to result in a live birth. We will review the link between age, genetics, and increased risk of miscarriage in Chapter 4.

Paternal age and increased risk of miscarriage is just starting to be an area of focus in research. Advanced reproductive age in men can be associated with increased risk of miscarriage. One meta-analysis pooling data from 10 population-based studies showed paternal age beyond age 40 to be significantly associated with an increased risk of miscarriage, adjusted for maternal age.[10] This is an important area of research to follow.

Risk of Recurrent Miscarriage

It's estimated that only 5% of women will experience two or more miscarriages and less than 1% of women will experience three or more miscarriages.[11] The risk of miscarriage increases with history of previous miscarriages and with age. The chance of miscarriage with a first pregnancy is 11-13% and increases to 14-21% after one miscarriage, 24-29% after two miscarriages, and 31-33% after three miscarriages.[11]

These numbers can be uncomfortable to hear, so remember, miscarriage is common, but so is having a baby. In one study looking at chances of miscarriage at different ages and number of previous miscarriages, researchers found that a 35-year-old woman with a history of five miscarriages still has a 62% chance of having a baby with her very next pregnancy.[12] Patients in the middle of their struggle with miscarriage can feel like their chance of miscarriage on their next try is 100%, but the statistics and studies show that this is just not the case.

> Every pregnancy is a new opportunity. Most women with miscarriage have a higher chance of having a live birth with their next pregnancy than another miscarriage. Many patients don't feel this way, but the research and data support it!

I want my patients to have a realistic understanding of their chances of another miscarriage, but I have many reasons to leave them feeling encouraged and positive. I want my patients to leave my office feeling educated, empowered, and encouraged to try to conceive again, either naturally or with treatment, and I want you to feel the same after reading this book. It's all about changing the mindset from feeling broken to feeling confident and cared for moving forward.

Key Points
- **Miscarriage** is a pregnancy that stops developing before viability.
- **Biochemical miscarriage** is a pregnancy loss before visualization on ultrasound or detection by histopathologic tissue diagnosis. A biochemical miscarriage is typically a positive urine or blood test for bHCG followed by a late menstrual period.
- **Clinical miscarriage** is a pregnancy loss after visualization on ultrasound or detection by histopathologic tissue diagnosis.

- **Recurrent pregnancy loss** is defined by ASRM as two or more miscarriages, regardless of how far along the pregnancy may be.
- Medical documentation of miscarriage can include the term **abortion** and can be confusing and even hurtful to patients who do not realize that the medical term abortion means the termination of a pregnancy before viability and does not include how or why the pregnancy ended.
- Miscarriages are common and occur in at least one in four clinically recognized pregnancies (incidence of miscarriage would be higher if biochemical miscarriages were included).
- Recurrent pregnancy loss is less common, and it's estimated that only 5% of women will experience two or more miscarriages and less than 1% of women will experience three or more miscarriages.
- The chance of miscarriage increases with age and number of previous miscarriages, but the chance of successful subsequent pregnancies remains high.

> **"Out of difficulties grow miracles."**
> – **Jean de La Bruyère**

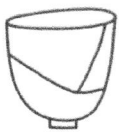

2

Why Me? Evaluation and Treatment of Recurrent Pregnancy Loss

Having a miscarriage can result in feelings of loss, sadness, and an intense desire to know why it happened. My patients tell me every day that they feel **broken**. They worry that they did something to cause their miscarriage, and they want answers so that they can prevent it from happening again. When you add another miscarriage, and another, these feelings pile up. Feelings of sadness and loss can turn to desperation, self-doubt, and fear regarding the inability to have the baby they desire. People want answers and solutions.

Some of my patients report going to appointments with questions and concerns regarding miscarriage and feeling dismissed by previous healthcare providers. They tell me that some doctors do not listen, do not offer testing, and shut down discussions about recurrent pregnancy loss (RPL). If this has been your experience, it's important to find a provider who will listen to you and at least discuss the option of testing with you. If you understand the tests for common causes of miscarriage, you will be able to have a deeper discussion with your provider and advocate for the care you wish to receive.

Do not be surprised if different providers order different tests or if you read conflicting recommendations on the internet. The field of reproduction, fertility, and especially miscarriage is evolving, and we're learning more every day. As we learn, recommendations change, and tests that were standard in the past are no longer considered helpful. Expert groups in women's health do not always agree on which tests should be ordered, so you can imagine providers will differ in their practice. Also, be careful what you read on the internet, because not everything is accurate or up to date with current understanding.

With ongoing research and increased knowledge, recommendations will change. In Chapter 3, we will review tests and treatment options for RPL that are controversial; but in this chapter, we will review the most common and expert-agreed-upon approach. Expert groups differ and will be noted, but the focus will be on recommendations from the American Society of Reproductive Medicine (ASRM), the expert group for recurrent first trimester miscarriage in the United States.

Common Causes of Miscarriage

The evaluation of RPL focuses on anatomic, genetic, immune, and hormonal issues that can be detected in the people who are conceiving; however, before I start testing, I warn patients that most often, the tests come back 'normal.' Hearing that we will most likely not find an answer for RPL can be frustrating for the couple, so it's very important to set expectations and explain why.

The most common cause of first trimester miscarriage is an issue in the embryo, not the people conceiving.[1] In first trimester miscarriages that are tested, 60-80% will have a genetic condition called a chromosome imbalance within the embryo that explains why the pregnancy stopped developing.[2,3] This chromosomal imbalance (also called **aneuploidy**) is unique to each pregnancy and in many ways bad luck, but also a natural part of reproduction. Miscarriage can be the body's recognition of a pregnancy that would not have been a healthy baby. This understanding does not take away the grief and feelings of loss with miscarriage, but it can help patients feel less '**broken**.' It doesn't feel like it, but women's bodies are often 'working correctly' when they miscarry.

> Before I order a single test for recurrent pregnancy loss, I set expectations that we will not likely find an answer. The testing for miscarriage focuses on issues in the people conceiving, but the most common cause of miscarriage is a chromosome imbalance (genetic issue) within the embryo.

Testing the <u>people</u> who are having miscarriages will NOT show genetic imbalances in the embryos that are miscarrying. The evaluation for RPL focuses on issues in the couple that may put them at risk for miscarriage. These are issues that may be 'fixed' and reduce the risk of a subsequent miscarriage.

We will review the anatomic, genetic, immune, and hormonal conditions associated with RPL and the tests used to discover them. By the end of the chapter, you should have a better understanding of not only the common causes of miscarriages, but the tests used to find them.

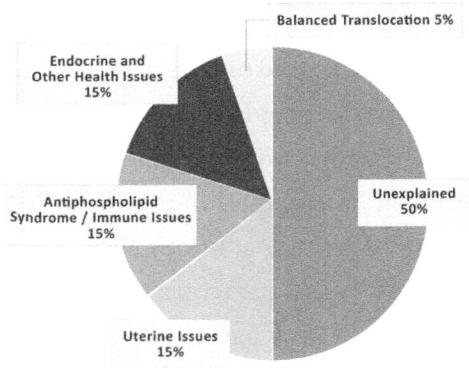

Causes and Incidence of RPL[1]

Not Broken

An Approachable Guide to Miscarriage and Recurrent Pregnancy Loss

Second Edition

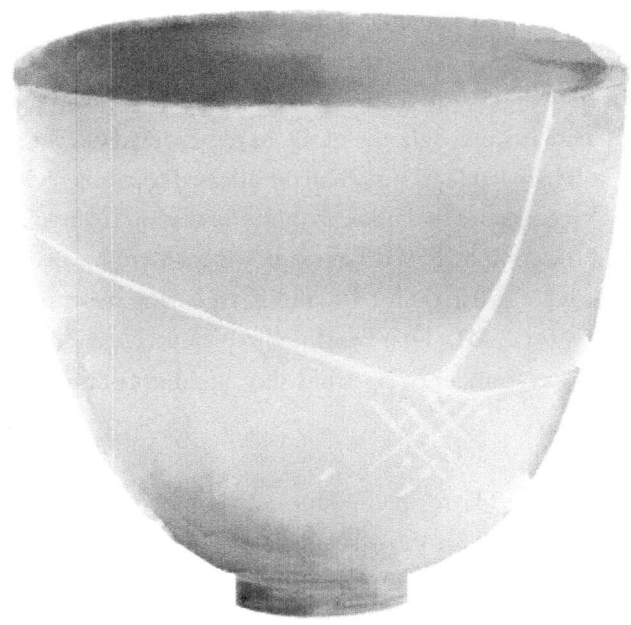

LORA SHAHINE, MD, FACOG

Seattle, Washington
2022

"Dr. Shahine has poured her vast expertise into this much-needed source of information for women and couples who have experienced miscarriage. She clearly explains Western medical treatments but also includes Chinese medicine principles and recommendations for lifestyle changes. Her approach is compassionate, supportive, and broadly informed. I highly recommend this book to anyone whose efforts to conceive have resulted in pregnancy loss."
– **Lynn Jensen, E-RYT, RPYT, MBA**, coauthor of *Yoga and Fertility: A Journey to Health and Healing*

"As both a fertility physician and a person who experienced multiple pregnancy losses, I am so thankful for *Not Broken*. Dr. Lora Shahine has compiled exactly what we all need – an approachable, evidence-based book to help guide patients through one of the hardest journeys. Her attention to detail while still being able to simplify complicated topics is truly spectacular. I recommend this book without hesitation to anyone wanting to understand the complexities of pregnancy loss and to have a resource for understanding what to ask their own physician during treatment."
– **Natalie Crawford, MD,** board certified reproductive endocrinology and infertility expert, cofounder of Fora Fertility, and host of the As a Woman Podcast

"I am so grateful to Dr. Lora Shahine for creating such an accessible and sensitively written book for those struggling with recurrent miscarriages. For women who aren't lucky enough to have her as their own physician, now they can at least empower themselves with the knowledge and practical tips necessary to work in tandem with their doctor to increase their odds of delivering a healthy baby."
– **Roohi Jeelani, MD,** director of research and education at VIOS Fertility Institute

work about a topic that, since the beginning of mankind, has been shrouded in emotions, guilt, and sorrow. Bravo!"
– **Paul J. Turek, MD, FACS, FRSM**, director of the Turek Clinics for men's reproductive health in Beverly Hills and San Francisco, master microsurgeon, and award-winning blogger, speaker, and author

"*Not Broken*, by Dr. Lora Shahine, is a truly essential, up-to-date guide to recurrent pregnancy loss. She explores the many causes of miscarriage and details a wide array of treatment options, ranging from high-tech medical interventions to lifestyle and wellness approaches. Dr. Shahine also addresses emotional health, making this book an essential companion that I would highly recommend to anyone traveling this path!"
– **Fiona McCulloch, BSc, ND**, author of *8 Steps to Reverse Your PCOS*

"I love this book! It's the resource you need during one of the most devastating times in your life. There aren't many things in the human experience more painful than living through pregnancy loss. When you have seen the spark of life and have it taken away, you become desperate for answers and look everywhere for hope. This book is exactly what my patients need because it explains things carefully and offers helpful tips and steps toward a healthy pregnancy. I highly recommend this book!!"
– **Aimee Eyvazzadeh, MD, MPH**, reproductive endocrinologist, fertility specialist, and patient advocate nationally known as "The Egg Whisperer"

"*Not Broken* is an essential read for any couple who has experienced a miscarriage. Dr. Shahine takes an emotional and complicated subject and breaks it down into an easy-to-understand format with hopeful and empowering advice. Dr. Shahine not only addresses the physical side of miscarriage but the psychological toll as well. She offers both Western and Eastern approaches to minimize a patient's risk of miscarriage. This will be a recommended read for all my patients who have suffered the loss of a pregnancy."
– **Peter G. Harvey, LAc, MSOM, FABORM**, of Eastern Healing, Inc.

Praise for Not Broken: An Approachable Guide to Miscarriage and Recurrent Pregnancy Loss

"I have one word to describe this fabulous book: finally. Women with recurrent pregnancy loss have been needing this book for years. Chock full of all the most up-to-date medical information as well as practical advice, this is a must-have resource for every woman and couple struggling for answers."
– **Alice D. Domar, PhD**, executive director of the Domar Centers for Mind/Body Health, director of Integrative Care at Boston IVF, senior staff psychologist in the Dept of OBGYN at Beth Israel Deaconess Medical Center, part-time associate professor of obstetrics, gynecology, and reproductive biology at Harvard Medical School, and author of *Conquering Infertility* and *Finding Calm for the Expectant Mom*

"I am so grateful to Dr. Lora Shahine for creating such an accessible and sensitively written book for those struggling with recurrent miscarriages. For women who aren't lucky enough to have her as their own physician, now they can at least empower themselves with the knowledge and practical tips necessary to work in tandem with their doctor to increase their odds of delivering a healthy baby."
– **Toni Weschler, MPH**, author of *Taking Charge of Your Fertility*

"This book is a very valuable resource for women who have experienced a pregnancy loss and are trying to make sense of what next steps they can take to build a family."
– **Judy Simon, MS, RDN**, registered dietitian and owner of Mind Body Nutrition, PLLC

"In her work, *Not Broken*, Dr. Shahine has surely 'broken' the mold of writing in typically cold, sterile medspeak to describe an intensely emotional issue in reproductive medicine: pregnancy loss. Indeed, she has written a demystified, finely tuned, understandable, and easily digestible

Chapter 2.1: Anatomic Issues, Tests, and Treatment

Up to 10-15% of women with RPL will have an anatomic issue that increases their risk of miscarriage.[1] These issues can be something the woman is born with, like a uterine septum, or an issue that develops over time, like a uterine fibroid. Uterine cavity evaluations like saline infusion sonogram or hysterosalpingogram can help diagnose an anatomic issue, and most are treated with a surgical procedure.

Uterine Anomalies

Uterine issues that women can be born with include a variety of findings called uterine anomalies and occur as the uterus is developing at its earliest stages. The uterus forms from two separate structures – two uteruses and two cervixes that come together as the fetus develops. An alteration in development during this process results in a uterine anomaly later in life. Uterine anomalies range from two totally separate uteruses and cervixes called a uterine didelphys (if the two structures never join) to a simple fibrous band of tissue in the middle of the uterus called a uterine septum (if the portion separating the two original structures never goes away).

It is difficult to estimate how common uterine anomalies are since many women go through life and have their children without miscarriages or without receiving imaging that shows the anomalies. Women with recurrent pregnancy loss likely have a higher incidence of uterine anomalies than women without recurrent pregnancy loss.[4] Not all uterine anomalies increase risk of miscarriage. Most experts agree that a uterine septum increases risk of miscarriage and should be removed in women with RPL while uterine didelphys should not be treated surgically. If you have a uterine anomaly, discuss your options with your doctor.

UTERINE ANOMALIES

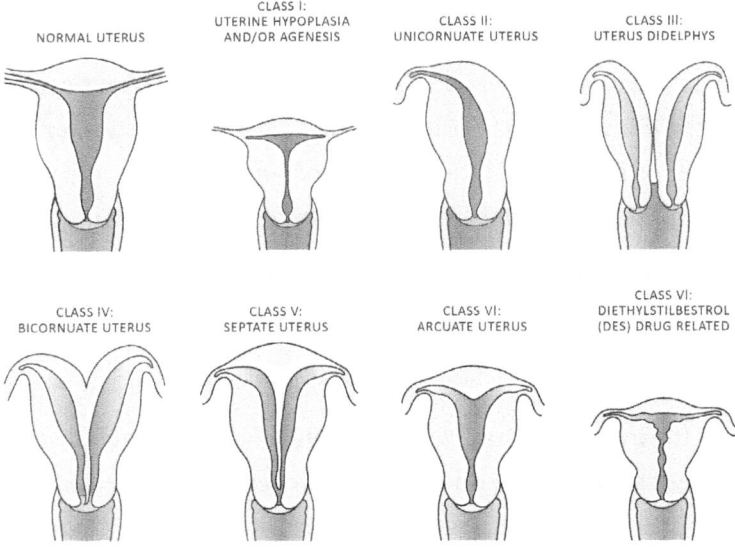

Other Uterine Issues

Uterine issues that may develop later in life include uterine fibroids, polyps, and adhesions or scarring. They can be diagnosed with similar imaging studies and often are treated with surgical procedures.

Fibroids

Fibroids are benign tumors made of fibrous tissue of the uterus and can be found in 40-50% of all women.[5] Some fibroids cause heavy bleeding, bladder pressure, and pain with menses, but many women with fibroids have no symptoms. Not all fibroids affect fertility, increase risk of miscarriage, or need to be removed.

The types of fibroids usually associated with miscarriage are either located within the uterine cavity where an embryo would implant or significantly large in size. Most experts agree that submucosal fibroids (located within the uterine cavity where an embryo would implant) impact embryo implantation and increase risk of miscarriage.[5] Submucosal fibroids can often be removed with a minimally invasive surgery called a hysteroscopy.

Many experts agree that most fibroids located outside the uterine cavity, within the wall of the uterus (called **intramural fibroids**) or located on the surface of the uterus (called **subserosal fibroids**), do not increase miscarriage risk. However, some experts argue that large fibroids (over 5-7cm) may increase risk of poor obstetric outcomes like preterm labor and increase risk of C-section no matter where they are located.[6] Your doctor will consider both location and size of fibroids when deciding on whether an intervention is right for you. Not all fibroids need to be treated, and removing fibroids unnecessarily may impact the function of the uterus and should be considered carefully.

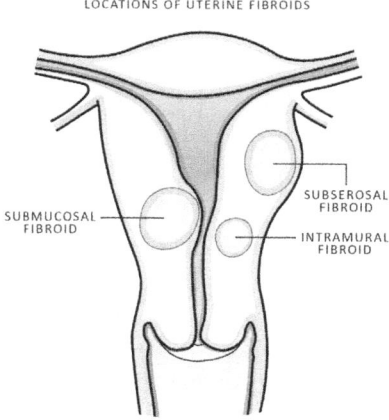

LOCATIONS OF UTERINE FIBROIDS

Polyps

Uterine polyps can be described as soft overgrowths of the uterine lining (endometrial tissue), like skin tags but in the uterine cavity. Some patients may experience spotting, but many do not have symptoms from polyps. They are often discovered during uterine cavity evaluations like ultrasound, saline infusion sonograms, and hysterosalpingograms. Most polyps are benign (not cancerous). Studies do not consistently show a direct correlation between uterine polyps and miscarriage, but some experts argue that they may impact embryo implantation. In fertility studies, the removal of polyps has been correlated with higher success with fertility treatment.[7] Experts do not agree on whether polyps increase risk of miscarriage, but many agree that they <u>may</u> and that the procedure to remove polyps (hysteroscopy) is very low risk. The potential benefit of polyp removal may outweigh the minimal risk of the procedure, but you should discuss your personal situation with your doctor.

Uterine Scarring and Adhesions

Uterine scarring may affect embryo implantation and increase risk of miscarriage. Uterine scarring (sometimes called **Asherman's syndrome** or intrauterine adhesions) is the presence of scar tissue in the uterine cavity, usually found after a uterine surgery or procedure and, rarely, after a significant pelvic infection involving the uterus.

Women with a history of procedures on the uterus (D&Cs) or intrauterine devices (IUDs) for contraception are often very worried about the potential effects on their uterus, but in most cases, these procedures have no impact on future reproduction. A sign of uterine adhesions can be a significant decrease in menstrual flow after a uterine procedure like a dilation and curettage (D&C). Menstrual bleeding can be light because adhesions can block the buildup of a thick uterine lining that can support a pregnancy, and the removal of these adhesions can repair the uterus, making it more receptive to embryo implantation. If you have noticed a significant decrease in days of bleeding or amount of menstrual flow after a D&C or uterine procedure, you should discuss the possibility of uterine adhesions with your doctor. Some women naturally have a light flow of menses; I usually look for a <u>change</u> in a woman's usual pattern after a procedure as a warning sign for scarring.

> Scarring after a D&C is extremely rare and is usually associated with a significant change in menstrual pattern and flow (much lighter) after the procedure. Uterine cavity evaluations like saline sonogram, hysterosalpingogram, or hysteroscopy will diagnose scarring, but I try to reassure patients that it is very rare.

Uterine adhesions can be treated with a hysteroscopy, a minimally invasive procedure in which a small hysteroscope is passed through the cervix to visualize and treat issues within the uterine cavity. It can be very scary to hear that there may be scarring in the uterine cavity, but I reassure patients every day that the uterus is a very forgiving organ – it is vascular (has lots of blood flow), heals well, and is designed to increase in size to accommodate a term pregnancy and then shrink back to its original size within weeks. Treatment of uterine adhesions results in a decreased risk of future miscarriage;[8] once the adhesions are removed and the uterus healed, most patients report returning to their previous menstrual flow and successfully conceive.

Imaging for Anatomic Issues

Imaging the uterus is the only way to know if someone has a uterine anomaly or uterine cavity issue. There are several options for imaging, including hysterosalpingogram (HSG), sonohystogram or saline infusion sonogram (SIS), magnetic resonance imaging (MRI of the pelvis), ultrasound of the pelvis including 3D ultrasound, and a hysteroscopy. Each test is described below.

The most common first tests to evaluate for a uterine issue are either the HSG or SIS. These tests evaluate the uterine cavity when it is distended with liquid. In its natural state, the uterine cavity walls are collapsed together – it takes the infusion of liquid into the cavity (like inflating a balloon with water) to distend it gently and allow the complete visualization and evaluation for uterine abnormalities. If the initial screening tests are reassuring, then the uterine cavity is considered normal. If the HSG or SIS is suspicious for an abnormality, then a more definitive test like a 3D ultrasound, MRI, or hysteroscopy is usually the next step.

Hysterosalpingogram (HSG)

Hystero (uterus) salpingo (tube) gram (study) is the evaluation of both the uterine cavity and fallopian tubes with contrast dye and fluoroscopy. During the 10 to 15-minute study, a patient lies on a table, usually in a radiology department in the 'pelvic exam' position. A speculum is placed in the vagina so that the cervix (bottom portion of the uterus and opening to the uterine cavity) can be seen clearly. A catheter (small tube) is placed in the cervix, and contrast dye (it's actually clear in color but looks dark on x-ray) is injected through the uterine cavity and through both fallopian tubes while fluoroscopy (X-rays) are taking images of the contrast dye flowing through the reproductive tract.

The exam can be crampy, and many providers recommend taking an over-the-counter medication like ibuprofen before the procedure to decrease discomfort. Many patients would rather be doing something else for those few minutes (obviously) but report that the test is not as bad as made out by many online blogs and reviews. It can be uncomfortable and crampy, but it is usually quick, and the cramps resolve quickly too. That being said, it can be quite uncomfortable for some people. Talk to your medical team about what to expect.

The technicians and providers doing the study will be wearing lead aprons because a small amount of radiation is used for the procedure. They wear it for protection because they do this procedure often, but your exposure is minimal (less exposure than a long airplane flight). Patients can still try to conceive in the cycle they do the HSG (unless their doctor recommends otherwise) because the procedure is usually timed before ovulation in the cycle.

Sonohystogram

Also called saline infusion sonogram or SIS, a sonohystogram is an evaluation of the uterine cavity that involves distending the cavity with sterile saline (saltwater) while doing a pelvic ultrasound. The patient assumes the pelvic exam position; a speculum is placed in the vagina so that the cervix (bottom portion of the uterus and opening to the uterine cavity) can be seen clearly. A catheter (small tube) is placed through the cervix, and while sterile saline is passed through the catheter to distend the uterine cavity, a transvaginal ultrasound (a wand with an ultrasound probe placed in the vagina) is used to take images of the uterine cavity. Talk to your medical team about what to expect that day for you.

HSG vs. SIS

The HSG and SIS can both screen for uterine cavity defects. The HSG will evaluate the status of the fallopian tubes and evaluate the inside of the uterus, but it will not image the outside of the uterus (it could miss fibroids outside the uterine cavity) or the ovaries (it could miss ovarian cysts). The SIS does not evaluate the fallopian tubes, but it does show the entire uterus (inside and out) and allows for a view of the ovaries to rule out ovarian cysts. You can discuss the pros and cons of each test with your doctor.

Other Imaging Tests for Anatomic Issues

The HSG and SIS can find most uterine cavity abnormalities, but additional testing may be required, especially to definitively diagnose uterine anomalies. These options include a pelvic MRI, 3D ultrasound, and a hysteroscopy. If the HSG or SIS show suspicion for a uterine anomaly, your provider will likely order an MRI or 3D ultrasound. Before pelvic MRI and 3D ultrasound became more accessible, patients would require a procedure with both hysteroscopy (camera inside the uterine cavity) and laparoscopy (camera through the belly button to see the top of the uterus) to fully diagnose uterine anomalies. Pelvic MRI and 3D ultrasound are a less invasive way to see the entire uterus (inside and out). They also allow for imaging of the kidney or renal system since uterine anomalies are often associated with a congenital kidney defect like missing one kidney.[9]

If the HSG or SIS show suspicion for uterine scarring, fibroids, or polyps, your provider will likely suggest a hysteroscopy. This minimally invasive procedure, in which a camera is placed through the cervix, can diagnose the presence of these defects and usually treat them at the same time.

In summary, the SIS or HSG is usually ordered first with a RPL evaluation; if these tests show a possible uterine abnormality, then a follow up test like a pelvic MRI or 3D ultrasound can be ordered. In some cases, the follow up test can be a hysteroscopy, which can not only clarify what the uterine abnormality is but sometimes treat it at the same time. Not all uterine abnormalities can be treated with hysteroscopy, but many uterine septums, submucosal fibroids, polyps, and uterine scarring can. Please discuss imaging options and treatment options with your doctor.

Treating Anatomic Issues

Treatment for uterine anatomic defects requires surgical intervention and should be considered carefully. Many uterine anatomic issues may be treated with a minimally invasive procedure called a **hysteroscopy** in which a small camera is passed through the cervix to allow visualization inside the uterine cavity.

Imagine that the uterus is a balloon and that the cervix (the bottom of the uterus) is the part of the balloon you use to fill it. The hysteroscope is passed through the cervix, and the camera on the tip of the scope shows the inside of the balloon or uterine cavity clearly. Fluid flows into the uterine cavity to keep it expanded, and with direct visualization, a small instrument can be passed into the cavity to fix the uterine issue.

> The pros and cons of surgical intervention for anatomic issues found during an evaluation of recurrent miscarriage should be reviewed thoroughly before proceeding with surgery.

Chapter 2.2: Genetic Issues, Tests, and Treatment

Balanced Translocation – One Genetic Issue in Miscarriage

The field of genetics is evolving, and we are learning more and more about the impact of genetics on reproduction every day. We've briefly discussed genetic issues in embryos (chromosomal imbalances) resulting in miscarriage (see Chapter 4 for a more thorough discussion on this), but there is a genetic issue in the people having miscarriages that can explain RPL. A **balanced translocation** is a genetic issue in a patient that can increase risk of miscarriage. This is a balanced exchange of material between two chromosomes that occurs at conception of the patient and results in increased risk of miscarriage for that person later in life. Although it is a rare cause of recurrent miscarriage (occurring in 3-5% of couples with three or more miscarriages), it can explain why a couple is having recurrent miscarriages.[1]

We need to go back to biology class for you to remember what a balanced translocation is, so take a deep breath and hang in there for a minute. Our genetic material (genes that code for every process in our body) is stored on chromosomes in our cells. Imagine a large stack of Legos® in which each gene is a Lego® and the entire stack (approximately 25,000 genes) is the chromosome. In every cell in our body, we have 23 chromosomes, and each chromosome has two copies (one copy from the egg we came from and one copy from the sperm we came from).

A person with a balanced translocation has all the genetic material they need to be a healthy, reproductive person, but back when the egg and sperm came together to make this person, an exchange of material occurred when the chromosomes met. A portion of one chromosome (say chromosome number 14) exchanged with another chromosome (say chromosome number 18). It was a clean break in chromosomes, and no genetic material was lost in this <u>balanced</u> translocation of the chromosomes. The resulting embryo, which becomes the adult who is trying to conceive, has all the genes and information they need to be a healthy adult. However, when that healthy adult tries to reproduce and the chromosomes do their matching, lining up, and separating, a high percentage of their eggs or sperm will be missing enough genetic material that the embryo they create will stop developing at some point, resulting in miscarriage.

BALANCED TRANSLOCATION

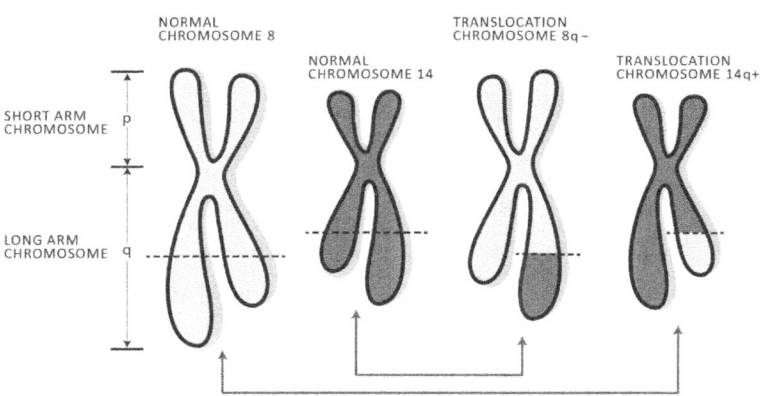

This does not mean that an adult with a balanced translocation is doomed to only miscarriages, since not all of their eggs or sperm will be affected. When a person with a balanced translocation tries to reproduce, three things can happen:
1. The resulting embryo will have a correct match of chromosomes and will likely result in a live birth.
2. The resulting embryo will have a balanced translocation just like the affected parent – with no effect on the development of the baby's health but a higher chance of having miscarriages as an adult.
3. The resulting embryo will have an unbalanced translocation, which usually results in a miscarriage but can also result in a baby who is born but has birth defects (because it is missing some genetic material). It is estimated that pregnancies with unbalanced translocation are born at term very rarely; only 0.8% of these pregnancies survive into the second trimester.[10]

A couple in which one parent has a balanced translocation can have a history of live births intermixed with multiple miscarriages.

Testing for Balanced Translocation

The test for a balanced translocation is called a **karyotype** and requires a blood sample. The cells in this blood sample are tested for their chromosome content, and balanced translocations can be found within one of the parents this way. The other way balanced translocations can be found is through testing the pregnancy tissue from a miscarriage – if this shows a balanced or unbalanced translocation, then both parents should be tested. One warning: there are different ways to test pregnancy tissue, and some labs will not be able to detect balanced translocations in pregnancy tissue. Another warning: the karyotype blood test can be costly, so it is important that your provider codes the test correctly and that you review with your insurance provider before testing.

Options for Patients With a Balanced Translocation

The treatment options for patients with a balanced translocation include either continuing to try naturally and hoping for the best or actively screening embryos for chromosomal abnormalities. Testing embryos before conceiving requires in vitro fertilization (IVF), which has its benefits but is high in cost and not always successful. In 2012, ASRM stated that evidence at that time did not support routine IVF with genetic screening of embryos for patients with RPL due to balanced translocation.[1] Proponents for IVF for these couples argue that IVF success rates are higher now than ever before and that this intervention will decrease the risk of miscarriage as well as all the psychological and physical burdens that can come with repeated miscarriages. Genetic counseling and a team approach are important if you test positive for a balanced translocation. The type of translocation will determine chances of success with either option, and a thorough discussion with your doctor is needed to help you make the best decision for you.

> Many doctors still do not test for a balanced translocation in their patients with recurrent miscarriage, arguing it is a high-cost test with low chances of being abnormal and may not change the patients' treatment path toward parenthood. I offer this testing to all my recurrent miscarriage patients because it is recommended by ASRM, knowledge is powerful for decision-making, and understanding why miscarriages are happening is beneficial for healing.

> **Patient Story**
> A young couple came to see me after years of trying to build their family. They had one young daughter and 10 miscarriages (some early biochemical losses and some first trimester losses), and I was

> a fifth or sixth opinion. They came with stacks of records – "We've been tested for everything, Dr. Shahine, I know there's nothing left, but we heard you specialized in recurrent miscarriage and wanted you to look at our case." I went through every lab test but could not find a karyotype for the patients – the young couple had been told by so many doctors that 'everything had been tested for' – they were sure they had done it but agreed to get the test done with my office. When I called to tell them the result (one of them did indeed have a balanced translocation), they broke down in tears. Tears of relief of a diagnosis, but also tears of fear – they had had a positive pregnancy test that morning. "Here we go again, Dr. Shahine, another miscarriage for sure. We'll do IVF with genetic screening of embryos next time, Dr. Shahine – I just can't have another miscarriage." This sweet couple went on to have a beautiful second daughter nine months later without IVF (just like their first daughter). I still get holiday cards from the couple with sweet messages like, "Thank you for all you did." I really didn't 'do' much for them, but I didn't assume all the tests had been done, and we did ultimately find the answer they were searching for all those years.

Chapter 2.3: Immune Issues, Tests, and Treatment

Antiphospholipid Syndrome (APS)

Many patients with miscarriage worry about immune and blood clotting issues. The one immune issue that is consistently screened for and associated with miscarriage and blood clotting is antiphospholipid syndrome (APS). APS is an **acquired thrombophilia**, meaning a tendency toward blood clots that is acquired – not inherited through genetic mutations. Diagnosis requires <u>both</u> abnormal blood tests <u>and</u> patient history of venothrombosis (blood clots in veins) and/or pregnancy complications. The presence of these antibodies in the first trimester may disrupt the process of placentation (the placenta implanting into the uterine lining), which may result in first trimester miscarriage or later poor obstetric outcomes due to poor placental function like preeclampsia, intrauterine growth restriction, and still birth. It's complicated and important to review.

Risk Factors for APS

The risk factors associated with APS are three first trimester clinical miscarriages (not biochemical miscarriages), one pregnancy loss after 10 weeks' gestation, and/or late obstetric issues associated with placental dysfunction like preeclampsia (a pregnancy complication associated with high blood pressure and other issues) or growth issues of the baby (like intrauterine growth restriction). One key point is that the timing of a pregnancy loss is based on when the pregnancy stopped developing, not necessarily the gestational age, since these can be different. For example, when an ultrasound shows that a pregnancy stopped developing at six weeks in size, the miscarriage occurred at six weeks, even if this is not diagnosed until 10-12 weeks' gestation. When reviewing patients' obstetric history, I always ask when the miscarriage was diagnosed and if an ultrasound was done. Very often patients tell me the miscarriage occurred at 10 weeks' gestation but that the ultrasound showed the fetus stopped developing at six weeks, measuring the size (see earlier discussion in Chapter 1 for more information on the importance of gestational age at time of miscarriage).

Diagnosing Antiphospholipid Syndrome

The diagnosis of antiphospholipid syndrome (APS) requires one of the clinical issues described above plus blood testing for the presence of antiphospholipid antibodies twice with 12 weeks between testing and at least six weeks since a miscarriage. The criteria for this diagnosis are very strict. No test is perfect, and the testing for these antibodies can be falsely positive from cross reactions with other antibodies. So in order to get a diagnosis, the test has to be positive twice, with 12 weeks between testing. It would be nice if the testing was black and white – positive or negative – but that's just not the way it is. ASRM recommends the following tests for APS:

1. Lupus anticoagulant
2. Anticardiolipin antibodies: IgG and IgM
3. Beta-2-glycoprotein I antibodies: IgG and IgM

There are other tests for this syndrome, such as screening for antiphosphatidylserine, but ASRM warns that the tests for other antibodies such as these are not standardized, and the level of evidence does not warrant routine screening.[1]

Treating APS

ASRM states that the standard treatment for patients who meet the above criteria for APS is low-dose aspirin and heparin.[1] Evidence shows a significantly higher live birth rate in patients using both medications compared to using aspirin alone.[11] **Aspirin** at a daily low dose of 81mg (sometimes called baby aspirin because the regular aspirin dose is over 300mg) decreases the risk of blood clots by making platelets in the blood less sticky. **Heparin** is a daily (sometimes twice a day) subcutaneous (meaning a tiny needle placed under the skin) injection medication that decreases risk of blood clots and directly decreases the presence of antiphospholipid antibodies. Heparin comes in two forms: unfractionated heparin and fractionated heparin (called **Lovenox**®). The traditional treatment for APS is aspirin at 81mg daily plus unfractionated heparin twice a day, but providers often use Lovenox® instead due to its once-a-day dosing. ASRM states that studies have not shown that Lovenox® is comparable to unfractionated heparin in the treatment of APS, but proponents of Lovenox® argue that the studies have not been done and once-a-day dosing of Lovenox® increases patient compliance.

In November 2017, ESHRE (The European Society of Human Reproduction and Embryology) updated their Guideline for RPL. The treatment of APS for patients with RPL remains controversial and the evidence conflicting. They conclude from all the evidence available to them at that time that patients with APS and RPL should be treated with low dose aspirin (75-100mg/day) starting before conception with a prophylactic dose of heparin (either unfractionated heparin or low molecular weight heparin (Lovenox®)) with a positive pregnancy test and throughout pregnancy.

Steroids for APS

Prednisone and other steroids are immunosuppressants and have been proposed as treatment options for APS, but both the 2012 ASRM and the 2017 ESHRE guidelines state that prednisone does not improve pregnancy rates in RPL patients with APS.[12] Both professional medical recommendations cite increased risk of premature delivery, neonatal intensive care unit admission, rate of preeclampsia and hypertension, risk of gestational diabetes, and lower birthweight seen in a 2005 study using prednisone in this population.[13]

IVIG for APS

IVIG (intravenous immunoglobulin) is an immune therapy proposed by some as a treatment for RPL related to APS. IVIG is a blood product prepared by combining serum from over 1,000 blood donors to treat patients with antibody deficiencies and diseases like Guillain-Barré syndrome and myasthenia gravis. Three randomized controlled trials (the best type of evidence available) showed NO improvement in outcomes in women with APS treated with intravenous immunoglobulin.[13] See Chapter 3 for more about IVIG as a controversial treatment option for RPL.

> **Patient Story**
>
> A couple came to see me after moving to Seattle from Australia for jobs in tech. They had been struggling to start their family in Australia and had been seeing a fertility specialist there for recurrent miscarriage before their move. They felt like they were at the end of their rope. She had one slightly elevated anticardiolipin antibody level during her work up, but it was negative when repeatedly checked. Since no other cause could be found, the doctor recommended full treatment for APS, which in his clinic meant aspirin, heparin, high dose prednisone, and IVIG infusions. She disliked the side effects of prednisone (weight gain and difficulty sleeping), but she was somewhat relieved to have a diagnosis and treatment plan. Unfortunately, the couple had two more biochemical miscarriages with this intense treatment regimen. I rechecked labs, could not find any evidence of APS, and asked them to rethink their current regimen. I was honest up front and stated I would not prescribe the same medications they had in Australia due to risks. They were nervous to proceed, but with their first embryo transfer (of a genetically screened embryo), we used our standard protocol <u>without</u> prednisone, heparin, or IVIG, and they had a beautiful baby boy. It's comforting to take medications – to 'do something,' but unnecessary treatment can come with risks, and all options should be reviewed carefully.

Long-Term Implications for APS

Diagnosis of APS may have implications for health beyond pregnancy. Being a reproductive endocrinologist means that I focus on helping people conceive and decrease the risk of a first trimester miscarriage. This means that patients move to another provider for obstetric care after the first trimester. Part of preconception counseling is building a care team for the patients. If a patient has APS, I refer them for a preconception visit with a high-risk obstetric provider who can help them with a care plan for medications throughout the pregnancy and often a hematologist who can advise them for care after pregnancy.

Chapter 2.4: Hormonal Issues, Tests, and Treatment

Hormonal Issues and Miscarriage

The hormonal issues associated with miscarriage include thyroid disorders, high prolactin levels, diabetes, and polycystic ovarian syndrome. The association of these endocrine issues with miscarriage can be debated among experts, like many issues in RPL, but screening includes simple blood tests, and treatment may decrease risk of another miscarriage.

Thyroid Dysfunction and Miscarriage

The thyroid is a butterfly-shaped gland that sits in the front of the neck and makes thyroid hormones. Thyroid hormones are responsible for many biological processes in the body, and disorders of the thyroid are associated with varying symptoms and problems. Miscarriage can be associated with both hyperthyroidism (the thyroid gland making too much thyroid hormone) and hypothyroidism (the thyroid gland making too little thyroid hormone).

Hyperthyroidism (making too much thyroid hormone, often referred to as Graves' disease) is less common and is treated with medication to control symptoms such as heart palpitations and to decrease the production of thyroid hormone. Untreated hyperthyroidism in pregnancy has been associated with increased risk of miscarriage, preeclampsia, preterm delivery, and congestive heart failure.[14] An endocrinologist specializing in thyroid care is usually the best doctor to manage hyperthyroidism and treatment before trying to conceive.

Hypothyroidism (low thyroid function) is much more common, and most evidence linking miscarriage to thyroid dysfunction involves low thyroid production. The fetus does not make its own thyroid hormone until approximately 10-13 weeks' gestation, so for the first trimester of pregnancy, the mother's thyroid gland needs to produce approximately 30% more thyroid hormone to make enough for herself and the baby. Hypothyroidism is associated with several poor obstetric outcomes, including preterm labor, lower IQ points in the baby, preeclampsia, and miscarriage.

The best **screening test for thyroid function** is TSH (thyroid-stimulating hormone), which is the hormone secreted from the pituitary gland underneath the brain that stimulates the release of thyroid hormone from the thyroid gland in the neck. It makes more logical sense to test the actual thyroid hormone levels, but the assay for these levels is less reliable (especially in pregnancy), which means that thyroid hormone levels in the blood do not always reflect what's really going on in the thyroid gland. If the thyroid is not producing enough thyroid hormone, then the TSH level will be high (the pituitary gland is pumping out TSH to get the thyroid to work properly). So, someone with a <u>high</u> TSH is <u>hypo</u>thyroid (counterintuitive, but that's how it works). The levels of the thyroid hormones (there are two: triiodothyronine or T3 and thyroxine or T4) are sometimes checked in conjunction with TSH to help define the issue and guide treatment.

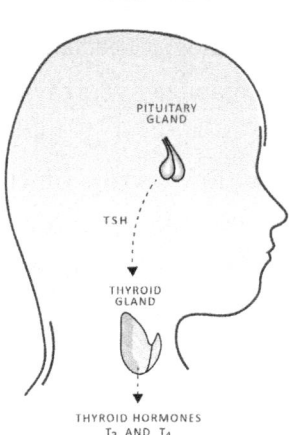

There is some debate as to which level of TSH to start treatment for hypothyroidism. In many labs, a TSH is labeled as 'normal' between 0.5-4.0mIU/L. However, many clinicians argue for a tighter control of thyroid function in patients trying to conceive (especially those with a history of recurrent miscarriage) due to the evidence that underactive thyroid is associated with poor obstetric outcomes. Providers may start treatment with thyroid hormone replacement medication if the TSH is over 2.5mIU/L in women who are trying to conceive or have a history of miscarriages, but this recommendation is debated.[14]

The most common cause of hypothyroidism is Hashimoto's disease or Hashimoto's thyroiditis, a condition in which the immune system attacks the thyroid, causing low production of thyroid hormone. If someone is diagnosed with hypothyroidism, blood tests that are positive for thyroid antibodies give a clue that it's an immune system issue causing the thyroid dysfunction. Some studies have found that patients with RPL can have elevated thyroid antibodies (specifically thyroid peroxidase or TPO antibodies) with normal TSH and thyroid hormone levels. Some providers treat RPL patients with positive thyroid antibodies with low-dose thyroid hormone replacement, but this has not been shown to be helpful in clinical trials and remains controversial.

Subclinical hypothyroidism (SCH) is a controversial topic. In this condition, the TSH levels are increased, but the thyroid hormone levels (T3 and T4) measure in the normal range. Some women may have symptoms of hypothyroidism, but most do not. Recommendations for treatment of subclinical hypothyroidism vary greatly among professional medical societies. The American Thyroid Association recommends levothyroxine (thyroid hormone replacement) treatment for pregnant women with SCH (TSH above trimester-specific ranges) and TPO antibody positive or SCH (with TSH levels above 10mU/L) and recommends considering treatment for pregnant women with TSH levels >2.5mU/L and TPO antibodies, or TSH >10mU/L. They do not recommend treatment for women with normal TSH and negative TPO antibodies.[15] The European Thyroid Association Guidelines for the Management of Subclinical Hypothyroidism in Pregnancy and in Children recommend treating SCH before conception and during pregnancy with levothyroxine.[16] The two studies noted in the recommendation treated to a TSH level <2.5mU/L.

ASRM updated their definition of miscarriage and recurrent pregnancy loss in 2020 but has not updated their RPL treatment guidelines since 2012. The 2012 treatment guideline states that women with RPL should be evaluated for thyroid dysfunction and acknowledge the varying guidelines and recommendations for treatments. The guideline simply states:

> "As long as thyroid-stimulating hormone (TSH) levels are in the normal range, there is insufficient evidence to recommend routine thyroxine (T4) testing or screening for anti-thyroid antibodies. However, this is problematic given the lack of consensus regarding the definition of a normal upper limit of TSH. Whereas TSH values of 4.0–5.0 mIU/L

were once considered normal, a consensus is emerging that TSH values above 2.5 mIU/L are outside the normal range."

The most recent update on caring for patients with RPL from ESHRE in 2017 reviews the evidence and states there is a "clear association between thyroid autoimmunity and recurrent miscarriage." They recommend testing TSH and TPO (thyroid peroxidase antibodies) in women with two or more miscarriages.

In conclusion, recommendations for thyroid testing and treatment are not black and white – studies are small and professional guidelines vary. All professional medical societies recommend treating overt and symptomatic hypothyroidism, but recommendations vary significantly on subclinical hypothyroidism or isolated elevated thyroid antibodies. Individuals must discuss their personal situation with their doctor when it comes to treatment for thyroid issues in association with miscarriage risk. Don't be surprised if you get different recommendations from different providers.

Hyperprolactinemia and Miscarriage

Prolactin is a hormone produced by the pituitary gland (a small gland found at the base of the brain), and its primary function is to increase breast milk production while nursing. High levels of prolactin can interrupt normal ovulation cycles (eggs being released from the ovaries) and are the primary reason why menses do not usually return to regular cycles until months after delivery of a baby. By disrupting ovulation while nursing, prolactin can be considered nature's way of spacing out pregnancies.

Prolactin can be produced by cells in the pituitary gland outside of nursing and cause symptoms like nipple discharge and irregular menstrual cycles due to irregular ovulation. Some women can have regular cycles but still have high levels of prolactin. High prolactin levels can be associated with miscarriage if ovulation is disrupted or implantation is affected in the second half or luteal phase of the cycle.

Screening for high prolactin levels requires a simple blood test. Providers will often repeat the prolactin test before starting treatment and recommend no intercourse or breast stimulation for 24 hours before the repeat test since these actions can temporarily elevate prolactin levels slightly and give a false positive result. If the prolactin level is consistently high, your provider may recommend imaging your pituitary gland to rule out any other cause for the high prolactin. The pituitary sits underneath the brain in the back of the skull, and imaging could show a growth or lesion pressing on the pituitary gland, stimulating the release of the hormone. No need to worry since the imaging (commonly an MRI) most commonly shows nothing or a very small collection of cells in the pituitary gland making the prolactin called a **microadenoma**, which can be treated medically. Experts debate when imaging should be done since it so rarely finds anything abnormal. Some argue imaging should only be ordered if a patient has symptoms like headaches or vision changes or if the prolactin level is significantly elevated.

High prolactin levels are treated with a medication called a dopamine agonist (usually bromocriptine or cabergoline). Normalization of prolactin levels with medication will decrease miscarriage risk for patients with a history of RPL.[17] These medications work very quickly to reduce prolactin levels, and patients who have had symptoms like irregular cycles can see their cycles become more regular quickly. The most common side effects are nausea and dizziness, and they usually resolve in a few days, but if they do not, you can try taking the pills at night to sleep through side effects or place the pills vaginally. What? Yes – I said vaginally – it still gets reabsorbed, and usually side effects go away. If any side effects do occur, they should be reviewed with your doctor.

It should be noted that experts disagree about screening for prolactin levels in asymptomatic women with RPL. The 2012 ASRM guidelines for RPL care note small studies that show lower miscarriage rates in women with hyperprolactinemia and RPL after treatment of the prolactin levels. The most recent ESHRE guidelines for treatment of RPL from 2017 review more data and state that prolactin screening is not recommended for women with RPL with regular menstrual cycles. Once again, review your personal situation with your doctor to decide the right testing and treatment for you.

Diabetes and Miscarriage

Consistently elevated blood sugars found with uncontrolled diabetes can be associated with increased risk of miscarriage.[18] A simple screening test for diabetes is a hemoglobin A1c (HbA1c), which is a blood test that shows the blood sugar control over the last three months. In many labs, a hemoglobin A1c of 5.6% or less is considered normal while over 6.5% can signal diabetes. A result between 5.7% and 6.4% can be a warning sign that blood sugar levels are high and that lifestyle changes such as diet and exercise may be needed. Uncontrolled diabetes is associated with miscarriage, but once blood sugar levels normalize, either with lifestyle changes or medication, a person's miscarriage risk is similar to someone without diabetes.[18] Intermediately, HbA1c levels less than 6.5% are not proven to be associated with increased miscarriage risk, but they can be a warning sign to improve one's overall health.

PCOS and Miscarriage

Polycystic ovarian syndrome (PCOS) is a common hormonal condition associated with different signs and symptoms that may or may not be related to an increased risk of miscarriage. Approximately one in ten reproductive age women suffer from PCOS, in which an imbalance of hormones can be associated with irregular menses due to ovulatory dysfunction, weight gain most often associated with insulin resistance, and signs of elevated male hormones like acne and hair issues (either thick, centrally located hairs like on the upper lip and chin or male-patterned hair loss like balding). The multiple symptoms and varied presentation of PCOS make it difficult to diagnose, and many women can go for years without knowing they have the condition.

Professional medical societies differ, but the most commonly agreed upon criteria for diagnosing PCOS is called the Rotterdam criteria (because that's where the meeting was held to decide this definition in 2003).

Rotterdam criteria: PCOS is diagnosed if a patient has two of the following three criteria:

1. **Oligoovulation** – Meaning irregular menstrual cycles due to ovulation dysfunction. This means unpredictable periods coming as often as every two weeks or as little as every few months due to a hormonal miscommunication.
2. **Excess androgen activity** – Meaning high levels of male hormones seen either physically or in blood tests. Women have both female hormones (like estrogen) and male hormones (like testosterone), and if women have a higher than usual level of male hormones, they can have physical signs such as acne and extra hair growth. These hormone levels can be tested in the blood as well.
3. **Polycystic-appearing ovaries on ultrasound** – Meaning either a higher than normal number of resting follicles (fluid-filled sacs within the ovaries that contain eggs) or a higher than usual size or volume of the overall ovary. I tell patients all the time that we should rename PCOS to poly-follicular syndrome or poly-egg syndrome. The word 'cyst' simply means any fluid-filled collection in the body, but people associate the word 'cyst' with disease and other bad

things. Follicles are 'normal' fluid-filled collections or cysts that contain eggs that are getting ready to ovulate. A follicle is a 'normal' cyst, and someone with PCOS just has too many of them. Sometimes people with PCOS get ovarian cysts just like anyone else, but this is different from the high number of follicles that lead to the definition and diagnosis of PCOS.

Whether PCOS is a risk factor for miscarriage is debatable. Some small studies suggest that women with PCOS have a higher chance of miscarriage[19] while other studies suggest that having PCOS does not increase risk of having RPL.[20] There are several aspects to PCOS that may put someone with PCOS at higher risk of miscarriage:

1. PCOS is associated with insulin resistance (including diabetes) and hormonal changes like elevated androgens (male hormones) that may impact egg quality and/or embryo implantation. Maybe patients with PCOS are undiagnosed diabetics and may be having miscarriages due to the consistently high blood sugars. Studies evaluating a link between insulin resistance, PCOS, and RPL have widely varying outcomes and no collective conclusions. Some studies using a medication called metformin to improve insulin function in PCOS patients with RPL showed improved outcomes in subsequent pregnancies,[21] while other studies showed no improvement with metformin.[22] A supplement called inositol has been used to improve insulin resistance in patients with PCOS – please review supplements with your doctor since supplements vary greatly and ingredients are not always what is presented on the label.
2. PCOS is associated with hormonal dysfunction. Maybe the hormonal changes associated with PCOS that impact ovulation as well could increase the risk of miscarriages due

to poor implantation or luteal phase issues. Some providers hope that inducing ovulation with medications like clomiphene (or Clomid®) and letrozole (or Femara®) will balance the hormonal environment and improve pregnancy outcomes. Both clomiphene and letrozole will improve chances of ovulation and help regulate menstrual cycles. With predictable and regular menstrual cycles, hormone levels become more balanced, and some argue that the luteal phase (the second half of the menstrual cycle after ovulation when the embryo implants) is improved. Research does not prove a decreased risk of miscarriage with these medications, but they will often help people with PCOS ovulate more regularly and decrease their time to pregnancy.
3. PCOS is associated with excess weight and obesity. Obesity increases the risk of miscarriage alone, and the cause is multifactorial. Patients with obesity and PCOS can see improvements in their symptoms like regulation of menstrual cycles and improved acne and hair growth issues with weight loss. One of the best first interventions for anyone with PCOS and obesity is weight loss in a safe, sustainable way, and this may decrease miscarriage risk as well.

There is no single treatment for miscarriage targeted at treating PCOS, and its association with increased miscarriage risk remains up for debate.

Patients with PCOS and RPL should be cared for carefully, without assumptions. These patients should have a thorough evaluation for RPL and not assume the miscarriages are solely due to PCOS. Evidence does not support routine use of interventions like metformin and inositol for all patients with PCOS and RPL, and each case should be examined carefully.

Chapter 2.5: Unexplained RPL

What About Unexplained RPL?

After a Western, evidence-based approach to testing for recurrent pregnancy loss, including anatomic evaluation of the uterine cavity and blood tests screening for balanced translocations, antiphospholipid syndrome, and endocrine disorders, approximately 50% of patients will still not have an answer as to why they are having miscarriages and will receive the diagnosis of **unexplained recurrent pregnancy loss**.[23,24] Many argue that this is because the testing is focused on the people conceiving, and that the most common cause of miscarriage is a genetic chromosomal imbalance in the embryo. This diagnosis is both a 'blessing and a curse' – it can be reassuring that no significant abnormality is found, but it can be frustrating to not have an answer after an evaluation.

Chromosome imbalances in an embryo are unique to each pregnancy, and many argue that the best approach is to just try again. This is exactly the advice many patients get from providers, which can leave them feeling disheartened, but it can be a positive approach to take. Some providers just say 'try again' without explaining why. If a genetic issue is unique to each pregnancy and the most common cause of miscarriage, then many unexplained RPL patients have a high chance that the next pregnancy will have the correct genetic make-up and will result in a successful pregnancy. The only treatment option available to decrease risk of conception with an embryo with a chromosomal imbalance is to screen the embryo before implantation, which requires IVF (in vitro fertilization).

Discussing all options for next steps is an important part of my counseling for patients with RPL. The benefits of trying naturally include less intervention and less cost, but the risks include the complications and time it takes to recover physically and emotionally from more miscarriages. The benefits of IVF with chromosomal screening are the decreased risk of miscarriage with a screened embryo and the reassurance to the couple that they have tried something definitive to avoid the grief and physical recovery from yet another miscarriage. However, IVF comes at a high cost and the potential of no success after a considerable effort. If IVF with chromosomal screening were free, easy, and a 100% guarantee of a healthy baby, many would jump at the chance, but IVF is not for everyone. A thorough discussion of each person's chance of success with this intervention is important before assuming it's the right choice for you. We will review this topic further in Chapter 4 on genetics.

For now, I hope you have learned about the common causes, tests, and treatment options available for patients with RPL. With this knowledge, I hope you can have a deeper discussion with your provider and be an advocate for yourself in your care.

Key Points
- Testing for recurrent pregnancy loss includes:
    1. Uterine cavity evaluation
    2. Patient and partner karyotypes
    3. Antiphospholipid syndrome testing
    4. Thyroid testing
    5. Prolactin testing
    6. Screening for diabetes
    7. Screening for PCOS
- Uterine abnormities can be evaluated with a saline infusion sonogram or hysterosalpingogram but may also require further imaging like a pelvic MRI, 3D ultrasound, or hysteroscopy.
- Genetics are important in miscarriage – the most common cause of first trimester miscarriage is a chromosomal imbalance in the embryo, and one genetic test for patients

with RPL is a karyotype looking for a balanced translocation in both partners.
- An immune issue closely associated with miscarriage risk is antiphospholipid syndrome, and diagnosis of this issue requires not only blood tests but specific clinical history.
- Hormonal issues associated with miscarriage include diabetes, thyroid dysfunction, high prolactin, and PCOS – recommendations for testing and treatment for these hormonal conditions vary among professional medical guidelines.
- The goal of testing is to find an issue that can be treated in the patients, but many times, most or even all of the tests come back without an answer.
- Patients with unexplained RPL have a high chance of being successful with their next pregnancy without intervention, and they should discuss all treatment options – including trying naturally and IVF with genetic screening of the embryos – with their doctors.

"Courage does not always roar.
Sometimes courage is the quiet voice at the end of the day saying, 'I will try again tomorrow.'"
– Mary Anne Radmacher

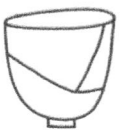

3

When Experts Disagree: Controversies in Care for Recurrent Pregnancy Loss

In Chapter 2, we reviewed the testing and treatment for recurrent pregnancy loss (RPL) that many providers and professional medical societies agree on. Now we will review the controversial issues surrounding the ever-changing field of miscarriage and RPL. Hang on, because this can be confusing, and different experts can get very passionate about what testing and treatment they believe in. You should see some of the debates at the medical conferences!

Unfortunately, not enough research focuses on miscarriage, recurrent pregnancy loss, and reproductive health compared to other areas of medicine like cancer and heart disease. A deficiency of well-funded scientific research to guide medical testing and treatment leaves a void for doctors to fill. Patients want answers, and their physicians want to provide them. Combine a lack of substantial scientific data with a vulnerable population of people appropriately desperate for answers, and you make room for interventions that may or may not work. Unfortunately, many of these medical interventions have risks, and patients must be aware of potential harm when undergoing any medical treatment.

> Patients have said, "I'll do anything to have a baby, Dr. Shahine, regardless of risk to me." It's my duty as a physician to do no harm

> and to thoroughly research any options. Patients can feel confused and stuck in the middle when I explain why I will not prescribe medications or do interventions recommended on the internet. I reassure my patients: we are all on the same team, we review every option, and we make decisions together.

While reading this chapter (and this book), please remember that we are still learning. There is very little black and white in the field of reproduction and miscarriage. Research takes time, resources, and people willing to participate in research studies. And when it comes to the field of reproduction, even when the resources are available, many studies cannot be done ethically because it's difficult to test new treatments on pregnant women – the stakes are too high if there are side effects and poor outcomes.

So, experts in RPL deal with the gray. It can be confusing at times for people with RPL desperate for answers when different providers tell them different things – and the internet can be either helpful or a rabbit hole of misinformation and confusion. Please remember to be patient with providers, who are trying their best, and do not believe everything you read on the internet, since things that sound too good to be true are most likely just that.

In this chapter, we'll review the causes and treatments for RPL that are controversial – the testing and treatment that providers may use but remain debated and not always supported by research and expert groups. I review important research studies, discuss professional medical guideline opinions when available, and will try to provide my own opinion when appropriate. The professional medical societies mentioned in this chapter include ASRM (American Society of Reproductive Medicine), ACOG (American College of Obstetricians and Gynecologists), RCOG (Royal College of Obstetricians and Gynecologist), and ESHRE (European Society of Human Reproduction and Embryology).

We will systematically discuss:
- Chapter 3.1: Blood clotting – testing and treatment controversies
    - Inherited thrombophilia like factor V Leiden
    - Methylenetetrahydrofolate reductase (MTHFR)
    - Aspirin
    - Heparin and Lovenox®
- Chapter 3.2: Hormonal issues – testing and treatment controversies
    - Luteal phase defect
    - Progesterone
    - Thyroid
- Chapter 3.3: Infection – testing and treatment controversies
    - Acute infections
    - Chronic endometritis or inflammation
- Chapter 3.4: Immune issues – testing controversies
    - Natural killer cells (NKC)
    - HLA typing
    - Cytokines
    - Thyroid peroxidase (TPO) antibodies
    - Antinuclear antibodies (ANA)
- Chapter 3.5: Immune issues – treatment controversies
    - Steroids
    - Intravenous immunoglobulin (IVIG)
    - Intravenous intralipids
    - Anti-tumor necrosis factor alpha (anti-TNF alpha)
    - Paternal leukocyte transfusion (aka lymphocyte immunization therapy)
    - Granulocyte colony-stimulating factor (G-CSF)
- Chapter 3.6: Genetic testing of miscarriages
- Chapter 3.7: Ovarian reserve testing

❏ Chapter 3.8: In vitro fertilization (IVF) with genetic screening of embryos as treatment for recurrent pregnancy loss

Chapter 3.1: Blood Clotting – Testing and Treatment Controversies

Inherited Thrombophilia

Patients are often worried about blood clots causing their miscarriage, but this is very rare. It makes logical sense that if the blood supply is compromised in a pregnancy, the pregnancy will stop developing, but this is very unlikely in early miscarriages. Pregnancy loss can occur later in pregnancy (especially in the second and third trimesters) when the blood supply in the placenta can be compromised by blood clots, but this is not typical in earlier miscarriages.

There is a mix of factors that make our blood more likely to clot (which is important to prevent excessive bleeding) or more likely not to clot (which is important in preventing blood clots that can lead to heart attacks and strokes). A defect in this delicate coagulation and anti-coagulation balance can lead to disease. Inherited thrombophilia is a genetic predisposition to making blood clots. This means that some people are born with genetic mutations that make them more prone to blood clots than people without certain genetic mutations. Inherited thrombophilia tests include factor V Leiden, prothrombin gene, antithrombin III, protein C, and protein S.

Please note that inherited thrombophilia is different from acquired thrombophilia due to antiphospholipid syndrome (APS) reviewed in Chapter 2. APS is an immune issue in which elevated levels of antibodies interfere with placenta implantation and function and result in multiple obstetric complications, including recurrent pregnancy loss. Please see Chapter 2 for more information on testing and treatment of acquired thrombophilia.

Pregnancy, and the high levels of estrogen associated with pregnancy, is considered a hypercoagulable state, meaning the coagulation balance shifts toward being more prone to blood clots. People with inherited thrombophilia can shift into blood clotting overdrive in a hypercoagulable state like pregnancy and have blood clots when other people would not. Some people (but not all) with inherited thrombophilia will have blood-clotting issues in pregnancy, like blood clots in the mother or blood clots in the placenta leading to intrauterine growth restriction in the baby or even stillbirth in the second and third trimesters.

In the past, routine evaluation for patients included testing women for inherited thrombophilia, but not anymore. Testing may be indicated if the woman has a personal or first degree relative with a history of blood clots, but not everyone with RPL needs testing for inherited thrombophilia. No professional medical society (ASRM, ACOG, RCOG, or ESHRE) recommends routine screening of RPL patients for inherited thrombophilia since studies do not show higher incidence of these issues in patients with RPL, and anticoagulation treatment in women with inherited thrombophilia and RPL does not decrease risk of miscarriage in a subsequent pregnancy.[1,2,3,4] Despite these clear guidelines, some doctors still order and act upon the tests.

Arguments for testing include:
1. Following earlier guidelines based on theoretical risks and limited research.
2. The desire to run all possible tests and provide patients with answers to why they are having miscarriages.

Arguments against testing include that:
1. Current evidence does not support an association between inherited thrombophilia and first trimester miscarriage.
2. Expert groups and guidelines do not recommend the testing.
3. Tests are expensive and a waste of resources.
4. Positive tests will likely lead to treatments and interventions that are not necessary and may cause unnecessary anxiety and harm (unnecessarily treating patients with anticoagulation or blood thinning medication when they do not need it).
5. Unnecessary treatment with anticoagulation medications has not been shown to improve the chances of having a baby.

In summary, some providers test for inherited thrombophilia, including factor V Leiden, prothrombin gene, antithrombin 3, protein C, and protein S, but the most current evidence and expert guidelines from multiple professional medical societies do not support this testing for a routine RPL evaluation. I do NOT order inherited thrombophilia testing on all RPL patients but take into consideration their personal, obstetric, and family history while deciding what is most appropriate for their care.

Methylenetetrahydrofolate Reductase (MTHFR)

MTHFR is an enzyme involved in multiple biological processes in the body. Some propose that mutations in the gene that codes for the MTHFR enzyme lead to dysfunction of this enzyme within the body that can lead to an increased risk of miscarriage. The proposed association of MTHFR gene mutations, MTHFR enzyme dysfunction, and miscarriage is one of the most heated disagreements among RPL providers, so let's learn a little more about MTHFR and what it does. MTHFR is involved in two main biological processes in the body: processing folate and converting homocysteine to methionine.

Folate is a B vitamin essential for many biological processes, including the production and maintenance of new cells, because it is integral in DNA synthesis. Some argue that miscarriage risk can increase if the body cannot metabolize and use folate properly in the creation of new cells in a developing pregnancy. Natural sources of folate include avocado, citrus fruits, beans, and leafy greens like spinach. Dietary folate must get converted in the body to be used in cells, and the last step in this process requires an enzyme produced with the MTHFR gene. Prenatal vitamins include folate (or folic acid) because women who have adequate folate levels during early pregnancy have a lower risk of having babies with neural tube defects like spina bifida.[5] **Folic acid** is a synthetic form of folate that is more easily absorbed and processed than dietary folates. 5-methyltetrahydrofolate (**5-MTHF**) is another synthetic form of folate that some claim is easier for the body to process than dietary folate, but this is debated.

Homocysteine is an amino acid and breakdown product of protein metabolism. High homocysteine levels have been associated with injury within blood vessels and a potentially higher risk of cardiovascular disease, blood clots, and miscarriages. MTHFR enzyme removes a methyl group from methionine to create homocysteine, and some argue that a mutation in the MTHFR gene will result in high levels of homocysteine. More recent evidence suggests that high homocysteine levels are a marker of risk of – not a direct cause of – blood clots.[6]

There are many mutations for the MTHFR gene, but the two most common ones are **C677T** and **A1298C**. When tested, people can be either heterozygous for these mutations (have a single mutation) or homozygous (have two mutations). In theory, the more mutations you carry, the more defective the MTHFR enzyme will be and the more health issues will arise.

MTHFR defects have been associated with many different diseases and health issues, from psychological disorders to cardiovascular disease to poor pregnancy outcomes. MTHFR mutations are extremely common, and 40% or more of people will test positive for a mutation in the MTHFR gene.[7] People who argue against testing point out that MTHFR mutations are extremely common (40% of the population) and RPL is not (<5% of the population), so it is unlikely that everyone with MTHFR mutations will be at increased risk of RPL.

Professional medical societies do NOT recommend testing for MTHFR mutations in patients with RPL. ASRM does not mention MTHFR in their 2012 guidelines for evaluation and treatment of patients with recurrent pregnancy loss.[3] The updated 2017 ESHRE RPL guidelines do not recommend testing RPL patients for MTHFR mutation.[4] Some providers do test for it and act upon the results.

Patients can feel stuck in the middle of providers making different claims about folate, folic acid, and MTHFR. Some providers suggest that taking a **prenatal vitamin with methylated folate** may compensate for MTHFR enzyme dysfunction in many people, but this is debated. Research supports taking folic acid to decrease the risk of neural tube defects.[5] ACOG recommends that pregnant women ingest a total of 600mcg of folic acid between diet and supplements each day.[8] More of something is not necessarily better or even good for you: too much folic acid can be associated with side effects like nausea, sleep dysfunction, and even seizures. However, patients with a history of pregnancies with neural tube defects are usually advised to take higher doses of folic acid in a subsequent pregnancy.

Check your prenatal vitamin for the type and dose of folic acid or folate listed and review options with your doctor.

Anticoagulation for Treatment of Unexplained RPL

Aspirin and heparin are two anticoagulation or 'blood thinning' medications used to treat and prevent blood clots. Anticoagulation therapy is recommended to decrease miscarriage risk in patients with RPL associated with acquired thrombophilia due to antiphospholipid syndrome (see Chapter 2 for more information on this), but what about these options for unexplained RPL?

Aspirin

Daily, low-dose aspirin has been used in women with recurrent miscarriages for decades, but the evidence supporting its benefits are varied. Aspirin not only decreases risk of blood clots by decreasing platelet aggregation, but it decreases inflammation by inhibiting the production of prostaglandins. Daily aspirin has been used in pregnancy to decrease risk of developing preeclampsia and other poor obstetric outcomes.[9] Aspirin has also been shown to increase uterine artery blood flow in women in the first trimester.[10] Some small studies show potential benefit, but larger studies and a meta-analysis of the studies available to date have not shown aspirin decreasing miscarriage risk for women with unexplained RPL.[11]

Proponents for aspirin use in RPL patients argue that risk is low in daily, low-dose aspirin, and that there may be a potential benefit, while proponents against the use of aspirin argue that there is no strong evidence that it helps, and it may increase risk of spotting and bleeding (but not miscarriage) in the first trimester. Aspirin can cause gastrointestinal upset and ulcers even at low doses. I discuss aspirin use with each of my RPL patients and review the pros and cons of its use – please review this option with your doctor.

Heparin

Heparin is an anticoagulation medication used in the prevention and treatment of blood clots that has been shown to decrease risk of miscarriage in patients with antiphospholipid syndrome (APS) and RPL. Heparin comes in two forms – unfractionated heparin that needs injections twice a day and low molecular weight heparin (Lovenox®) that requires once a day dosing. Three randomized controlled trials have studied use of heparin in patients with unexplained RPL and all differed in their design and findings. Two of the trials showed no benefit and one showed lower miscarriage rate with heparin. The trial that showed benefit included 300 patients with three or more unexplained miscarriages – 150 women received low molecular weight heparin through 20 weeks' gestation and 150 women did not.[12] The heparin-treated group had a higher live birth rate (73.3% vs. 48%). Risks of heparin use include pain at injection sites, bleeding, allergic reactions, and heparin-induced thrombocytopenia (low platelets). Professional medical societies do not recommend routine treatment of unexplained RPL with heparin, but some providers offer this option to patients.

> I review the risks and benefits of heparin and aspirin with my RPL patients. There are cases without clear answers, especially recurrent miscarriage with normal chromosome testing of the embryo, so I will sometime use aspirin and heparin. It takes careful counseling, and each case is unique.

Chapter 3.2: Hormonal Issues – Testing and Treatment Controversies

Luteal Phase Defect and Progesterone Treatment

The menstrual cycle has two phases: the follicular phase, which is the time between the start of a period and ovulation (the release of the egg from the ovary), and the luteal phase, which is the time after ovulation when an embryo can implant in the uterine lining. Embryo implantation is a delicate process involving hormone and immune interactions, and dysfunction in the luteal phase may play a role in increased risk of miscarriage. The controversies surrounding luteal phase defect and miscarriage involve both how to diagnose and how to treat the defect.

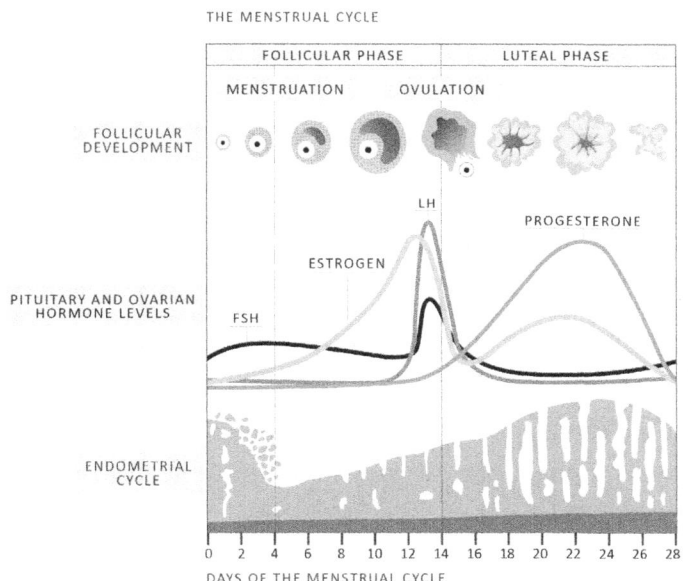

It makes logical sense that issues in the uterine lining and communication between the maternal system and the embryo in the luteal phase would impact the success of a pregnancy, but it's difficult to test for it and prove that there is even a deficiency to treat. There are tests that have been proposed to screen for luteal phase defect, including progesterone hormone blood tests and endometrial lining biopsies, but these tests have their faults.

Many RPL patients are worried about the link between progesterone levels and miscarriage – it's one of the most common questions patients ask. I'll review this issue more but will end the suspense and tell you now that:

1. I do NOT check progesterone blood levels unless I am trying to confirm ovulation.
2. I DO offer progesterone treatment to many patients with RPL.
3. I usually recommend starting progesterone supplements with a positive pregnancy test unless otherwise indicated.

If these three points surprise you and you've read differently or a provider has recommended something different, that's okay! Please remember that RPL is an evolving field, and we are constantly learning. I keep up with research and guidelines, and this is the course of action that seems to work best for most of my patients based on my current understanding.

More on progesterone and why it's so important: progesterone is the dominant hormone in the luteal phase, and it is made by the corpus luteum (the remaining follicle left over in the ovary after ovulation). Progesterone is essential for embryo implantation and support of early pregnancy until the placenta starts to make its own progesterone around eight weeks of pregnancy. We learned about the importance of the corpus luteum and progesterone from studies in the 1970s that showed that if the corpus luteum is removed before eight weeks' gestation (and therefore the only source of progesterone production is lost), then a miscarriage occurs. Why would anyone remove a corpus luteum, you ask? Sometimes during the release of the egg at ovulation, a blood vessel is disrupted, and bleeding occurs. If this bleeding is heavy, a person may need surgery to stop the bleeding. If the corpus luteum is removed or destroyed in order to stop the bleeding and the pregnant woman does not receive supplemental progesterone medication, then a miscarriage will occur.[13] If the corpus luteum is removed before eight weeks' gestation and a pregnant woman receives supplemental progesterone, then she is much less likely to miscarry.[13]

Progesterone may have many roles in implantation and support of an early pregnancy. Studies suggest that progesterone enhances uterine relaxation and allows the uterus to become more receptive to the embryo.[14,15] The immune interaction between the embryo and the uterine lining is delicate, and the uterine lining needs to accept the embryo (with some foreign genetic material) for successful implantation. Progesterone has a key role in the immune interaction and shifts the maternal immune system in the uterine lining to a more receptive state.[16] We're still learning, but progesterone is key for a successful early pregnancy.

Progesterone Deficiency Testing

Testing for a progesterone deficiency, either by blood tests or endometrial biopsies, has limitations. Patients often ask for progesterone levels by blood tests while trying to conceive or in early pregnancy, but these levels can be misleading. Progesterone is secreted by the corpus luteum sporadically, and one single blood test can either be falsely reassuring or falsely alarming, and the levels can be completely different a few hours later in the day. In addition, progesterone levels vary cycle to cycle, so levels in one cycle do not reflect what's happening in all menstrual cycles.

Testing the endometrial lining in the luteal phase for 'endometrial dating' was popular in the past but requires an uncomfortable endometrial biopsy and possible disruption of an early pregnancy, and it has also been shown to be inconsistent and unreliable.[17] ASRM's 2012 Guidelines for RPL state that luteal phase defect has been associated with pregnancy loss, but the assessment is problematic. Testing progesterone blood levels is not mentioned in the guidelines, and routine endometrial biopsy for diagnosing luteal phase defects is not recommended.[3] The updated 2017 ESHRE guidelines do not recommend testing for luteal phase defect with progesterone blood tests and/or endometrial biopsies.[4]

Progesterone Treatment for RPL

The importance of progesterone for successful implantation and maintenance of early pregnancy has led many physicians to prescribe progesterone supplementation for patients with RPL. A Cochrane review from 2013 with data from four small clinical trials concluded that progesterone supplementation in women with unexplained RPL decreased risk of a subsequent miscarriage, but critics railed against this conclusion given the small numbers of patients and the wide variation in design of each of the trials.[18]

In 2014, a double blind, placebo controlled, randomized trial[19] of oral dydrogesterone (not available in the US) for patients with unexplained recurrent pregnancy loss showed lower miscarriage rates in patients who received progesterone compared to patients who received a placebo. In this trial, 360 patients were randomly assigned to receive either 10mg of dydrogesterone twice daily or a placebo starting from four to eight weeks' gestation through 20 weeks' gestation. The group that received progesterone had a lower miscarriage rate (3.5%) compared to the placebo group (16.8%), and this finding was statistically significant ($P<0.01$). Critics of the study argue that including patients who start progesterone later than four to five weeks of pregnancy in the study alters the results, since clinically, most providers start progesterone earlier.

In 2015, a multicenter, double blind, placebo-controlled, randomized trial of vaginal progesterone for women with unexplained RPL showed no difference in live birth rates for women treated with progesterone vs. women treated with a placebo.[20] In this trial, 836 women were randomly assigned to receive either 400mg of micronized progesterone or a matched placebo pill from time of positive pregnancy test up to six weeks pregnant through 12 weeks of pregnancy. Live birth rate was 65.8% in the progesterone group and 63.3% in the placebo group. A randomized controlled trial is the ultimate scientific study because it should limit many variables – this trial should have answered the question about progesterone and miscarriage, but it has a big flaw. Progesterone likely has the most impact starting earlier in the pregnancy, so including patients who started treatment as late as six weeks of pregnancy leaves the conclusions in question.

A 2017 meta-analysis[21] pooled together data from multiple different trials looking at treatment outcomes in women with RPL and found a lower miscarriage rate in women who received progesterone compared to women who did not receive the progesterone. A problem with pooling data is that the trials are so different in type of progesterone given and the timing of dosing that the results are difficult to combine for one conclusion or single recommendation that fits every patient circumstance.

Professional medical guidelines do not support routine progesterone supplementation to women with RPL. ESHRE guidelines from 2017 review data available up to that date, some studies showing benefits of progesterone in women with unexplained RPL and others showing no benefit and conclude, "progesterone does not improve live birth rates in women with unexplained RPL."[4] Even though the evidence varies and professional guidelines do not recommend routine prescribing progesterone for RPL, many providers still prescribe it for their patients.

When to Start Progesterone Treatment

Another hot topic surrounding luteal phase defect and progesterone treatment for RPL is <u>when</u> to start treatment. Some providers recommend starting in the luteal phase (after ovulation but before a positive pregnancy test) while others start treatment only after a positive pregnancy test. Starting progesterone in the luteal phase is a more traditional approach, and a well-designed clinical trial in 2015 showed no benefit for progesterone supplementation in women with recurrent unexplained miscarriages when started after a positive pregnancy test.[20] Other studies have shown benefit to starting progesterone after pregnancy confirmation – including a meta-analysis in which 10 clinical trials were examined together to try to answer this question.[21] The decisions on if and when to start progesterone supplements should be discussed with your doctor.

In my practice, I offer progesterone to most RPL patients and usually recommend waiting to start progesterone until a positive pregnancy test in many cases for several reasons:

1. Some research supports that the benefits of progesterone in RPL are similar whether it is started in the luteal phase or after a positive pregnancy test.
2. If progesterone is started before ovulation, it may decrease the chances of implantation. The embryo and the uterine lining fit together like a jigsaw puzzle – a delicate communication exists between the hormonal and immune systems. In a menstrual cycle, the ovary makes estrogen to build up the uterine lining in the first half of the cycle, and after ovulation, the ovary makes progesterone to support the lining. If the uterine lining sees progesterone before ovulation (because someone takes a supplement too early), the uterine lining will be 'out of phase' or 'too advanced' and may not accept the embryo. If someone is taking progesterone before pregnancy, they need to be very sure they have ovulated before starting the progesterone.
3. Side effects of progesterone can be miserable for some people. Progesterone is the premenstrual hormone associated with bloating, mood swings, breast tenderness, fatigue, and more. Thorough counseling about what to expect, including the side effects of progesterone, is important.
4. There is an emotional impact involved in progesterone's ability to delay the onset of menses. The signal for the onset

of bleeding in a menstrual cycle is the decrease or absence of progesterone. For the two weeks after ovulation, the corpus luteum makes progesterone, but it stops making it unless a pregnancy producing bHCG (the pregnancy hormone) encourages it to continue making it. If there is no pregnancy and no bHCG to prompt the corpus luteum to make more progesterone, then progesterone levels drop and the uterine lining sheds. Taking progesterone supplements will delay this process and the start of a period will be delayed. Fast forward through the multiple home pregnancy tests with a missed expected day of menses and the frustration if the tests are negative. Supplemental progesterone will not prevent the start of a period forever, but it will delay it by a few agonizing days.

> Some patients worry about taking progesterone if it will prevent a miscarriage that was 'meant to be.' If I am prescribing progesterone, I remind patients that the most common cause of first trimester miscarriage is a genetic issue (chromosomal imbalance) in the embryo, and progesterone supplementation will not 'fix' that issue. Progesterone supplements will NOT stop a miscarriage from occurring if the embryo has a chromosomal imbalance.

In summary, progesterone may help some women with RPL. Furthermore, starting it with a positive pregnancy test may be as effective as starting it in the luteal phase, and there are several benefits to waiting. However, there are some cases where I start progesterone in the luteal phase. If women follow their cycles closely and they consistently have less than 10 days between ovulation and menses or they have luteal phase bleeding or spotting, I may recommend luteal phase progesterone. In these cases, I review the potential side effects and risks, benefits, and alternatives closely with my patients before we make that decision.

Options for progesterone supplements include intramuscular injections, vaginal suppositories, oral pills, and creams to rub into the skin. Intramuscular injections and vaginal suppositories have the most evidence to support benefit. Vaginal suppositories include creams and pills with applicators that are inserted into the vagina like tampons or pills patients place manually. Please review with your doctor whether progesterone supplements are right for you, and if so, which one is best for you.

Thyroid and Miscarriage

We reviewed testing and treatment of thyroid hormone abnormalities in Chapter 2, but we're re-visiting it here because many aspects for when to test and how to treat are controversial. For review, the thyroid is a butterfly-shaped gland in the neck that produces thyroid hormones, which are involved in many biological processes in the body. Both overactive (hyperthyroidism) and underactive (hypothyroidism) have been associated with poor obstetric outcomes, including miscarriage. Most providers agree on treating symptomatic thyroid disease and overt hypothyroidism to decrease risk of miscarriage, but providers and professional society guidelines differ in their opinions on who to test, when to treat, and more.

We reviewed tests for thyroid disease in Chapter 2, including thyroid-stimulating hormone (TSH), the thyroid hormones (T3 and T4), and thyroid antibodies. The best screening test for thyroid disease is TSH, and a high TSH can reflect an underactive thyroid gland (hypothyroidism). **Overt hypothyroidism** is a combination of a high TSH level with low thyroid hormone levels, and guidelines recommend treating women with overt hypothyroidism to decrease the risk of miscarriage.[3] **Subclinical hypothyroidism** (SCH) is a high TSH associated with normal levels of thyroid hormones, and most patients are not symptomatic. Evidence is conflicting regarding the association of SCH and miscarriage, and experts differ in opinion regarding who to test, how to define SCH, and when to treat. Debate also surrounds whether to test for and treat positive thyroid antibodies in the setting of no other abnormal thyroid tests in women with RPL.

Some experts recommend screening any women planning to conceive and starting treatment before conception while others recommend screening only in pregnancy. Some experts start thyroid replacement medication when the TSH is >4.0mIU/L while others recommend a tighter control and keep the TSH <2.5mIU/L. Some experts test and treat with positive thyroid peroxidase antibodies (TPO) with or without other abnormal thyroid tests. Experts against some of the testing argue that providers could be over-testing and over-treating without strong evidence to justify the increased costs, and experts for testing and treating argue that the treatment has minimal risk but potential benefit.

ASRM reviewed the current evidence for treatment of SCH in their practice guidelines in 2016.[22] They review not only the studies and controversies but report on the most recent consensus guidelines from the Endocrine Society, the American Thyroid Association, and the American Association of Clinical Endocrinologists.[23] It would be nice if all these experts could truly come to a consensus and just tell providers what to do, but even they still disagree on a few points.

ASRM summarizes thyroid testing and treatment for women with a history of miscarriages as follows:
1. It is reasonable to test TSH in women with a history of infertility and miscarriage before conception.

2. If TSH >4.0mIU/L, patients should be treated with thyroid replacement medication to maintain TSH levels at <2.5mIU/L.
3. If TSH is between 2.5–4.0mIU/L before pregnancy, options are to monitor or treat.
4. During the first trimester of pregnancy, it is advised to treat with TSH if >2.5mIU/L.
5. Thyroid antibody testing is not recommended routinely, but consider testing thyroid peroxidase antibodies when TSH >2.5mIU/L and consider treatment.

ESHRE's 2017 RPL Guidelines[4] state that overt hypothyroidism and hyperthyroidism should be treated before conception and closely through pregnancy when possible. The guidelines acknowledge the conflicting evidence regarding treatment of subclinical hypothyroidism but note that intervention may reduce the risk of subsequent miscarriage.

If the experts cannot agree on clear guidelines, you can imagine individual providers will have differences of opinion and practices. In my practice, I usually check TSH and thyroid peroxidase antibodies in patients with a history of recurrent pregnancy loss before conception. I treat to maintain a TSH <2.5mIU/mL at a minimum. I recheck TSH with a positive pregnancy test and recommend rechecking at least once a trimester in pregnancy. Thyroid needs go up once pregnancy occurs since the fetus does not make its own thyroid hormone until the end of the first trimester. Some providers will recommend increasing thyroid hormone medication with a positive pregnancy test. Please review thyroid testing and treatment with your doctor and weigh the pros and cons of all options in your discussion.

> When starting thyroid medication in patients with subclinical hypothyroidism and borderline TSH levels, I review that many providers would not recommend treating and openly discuss the controversies in recommendations. I review that thyroid function should be tested periodically while trying to conceive and multiple times in pregnancy since needs may change. Finally, I review that the majority of patients will not need thyroid medication after delivery of the baby but that the patient should review their care with their primary care doctor or obstetrician before stopping any medication.

Chapter 3.3: Infection – Testing and Treatment Controversies

Infection

Some bacterial and viral infections have been associated with sporadic but not recurrent miscarriages.[3] An **active infection** with *Ureaplasma urealyticum*, *Mycoplasma hominis*, chlamydia, *Listeria monocytogenes*, *Toxoplasma gondii*, rubella, cytomegalovirus, herpes virus, and other pathogens has been found in vaginal and cervical fluid from women with sporadic pregnancy losses, but these women are usually symptomatic with active illness.[24] Bacterial vaginosis has been associated with preterm labor later in pregnancy, but evidence for its association with first trimester miscarriage is inconsistent.[25] ASRM and ESHRE do not recommend routine screening for infections in asymptomatic women with recurrent pregnancy loss.[3,4]

Women who are pregnant are warned to avoid foods with high bacterial content like sushi, soft cheeses, and deli meat. This is due to the immune system being shifted in pregnancy and women being more susceptible to some pathogens than they would be outside of pregnancy. Pregnant women are more likely to get food poisoning, contract the common cold and flu (get your flu shot!), etc. These illnesses very rarely result in miscarriage, and these food warnings are cautionary.

Active infections are associated with symptoms like fever, body aches, vaginal discharge, and pelvic pain, but some providers screen for asymptomatic chronic uterine infection, also known as **chronic endometritis**. The theory is that a previous infection may have heightened the immune reactions in the uterine lining so that the active infection is resolved but embryo implantation is still adversely affected by leftover immune cells in the uterine lining. Experts debate on whether to test for and if so how to diagnose chronic endometritis, but proposed tests include either:

1. Hysteroscopy showing signs of inflammation (visualizing micropolyps or inflamed, red uterine lining seen through a hysteroscope placed through the cervix).
2. Microscopic detection of **plasma cells** (immune cells diagnostic of inflammation) from an endometrial biopsy using traditional hematoxylin and eosin (HE) staining.[26]
3. Microscopic detection of plasma cells (immune cells diagnostic of inflammation) from an endometrial biopsy using staining with **CD138**.[27]

An **endometrial biopsy** is a procedure in which a tissue sample from the uterine lining is obtained with a small, plastic, straw-like catheter passed through the cervix. The procedure is typically quick but crampy. The tissue is sent to a lab to evaluate for chronic inflammation, and if present, the patient is typically placed on a multi-week course of antibiotics. The physician doing the testing will discuss the different types of staining available (HE vs. CD138) with the pathologists and the lab who is doing the staining. Some argue that the CD138 testing is more accurate than the traditional HE staining and others argue they are similar.

There is no consensus on who to test, exactly what to screen for, or course of treatment if the tissue shows signs of inflammation, but some evidence shows poor outcomes in subsequent pregnancies if chronic endometritis is left untreated,[28] and other evidence shows resolution of inflammation if treated with antibiotics.[29] Some doctors will test for and treat chronic endometritis, but professional medical society guidelines do not support these interventions. The 2012 ASRM RPL guidelines do not mention screening for or treating chronic endometritis.[3] The 2017 ESHRE RPL guidelines[4] review some small clinical trials testing for and treating chronic endometritis in patients with RPL but conclude, "further research is needed including prospective observational studies and randomized controlled trials before screening women for endometritis can be recommended."

Arguments for testing for chronic endometritis are simple:
1. To find a cause for RPL and treat it.

Arguments against testing and treatment for chronic endometritis include that:
1. Testing is painful and costly.
2. There is strong evidence that testing for and treating presumed chronic endometritis does not exist.
3. Interventions, which are typically testing, treating with antibiotics for multiple weeks, and re-testing for a cure, are costly, time-consuming, and uncomfortable (including an endometrial biopsy) for the patient.
4. Interventions involve use of antibiotics for long periods of time, which may result in increased pathogen resistance to antibiotics and harmful impacts on the patient's microbiome.

In summary, research is ongoing regarding a link between chronic endometritis and recurrent miscarriage. In the meantime, the option of testing and the implications of retesting and long-term antibiotic exposure with its inherent risks should be discussed thoroughly with patients before testing.

> There are some instances when I test for chronic endometritis, but it's not a part of my routine evaluation of a patient with recurrent pregnancy loss at this time. I am wary of the potential harm and time lost in testing, treating, and retesting for a cure that is involved in this process without substantial evidence to support these interventions in all patients.

Chapter 3.4: Immune Issues – Testing Controversies

The Immune System and Immune Testing

One of the questions I ask patients when I meet them for the first time is, "What are you worried about?" I learn a lot about my patients and their concerns by just listening, and some of the most common worries for patients with RPL concern their immune system. I hear things like:

"I'm worried my body is attacking my babies."

"I'm worried that my body is attacking my partner's sperm."

"I'm worried that my body is not baby-friendly."

I start reassuring these patients right away. It is absolutely amazing that our bodies can accept 'foreign' genetic material and allow a baby to develop and grow inside of us! We know that our immune system keeps us safe from disease by attacking foreign viruses and bacteria, and in cases of organ transplants (carrying foreign genetic material inside), people take strong medication to suppress their immune system to not attack the 'new' material. We

know that some diseases like thyroid disorders a
arthritis result from dysfunction of our immune
sense to question the role of the immune system
implantation, pregnancy development, and recu

The role of the immune system in repro heated debate among experts. They agree that tl needs to adapt to allow embryo implantation, but that's where agreement ends. In the case of treatment for presumed immune dysfunction for miscarriage, the stakes are high, evidence supporting the efficacy of these treatments is weak, and results vary. Any treatment to suppress the immune system has the potential of causing harm and should be considered very carefully before starting. We'll review each group of immune issues, then discuss controversies in care.

Natural Killer Cells (NKC)

This is one of the most discussed and argued about tests for patients with RPL. Even though they have a terrifying name, natural killer cells are an essential part of the body's defense mechanism against disease. Some argue that dysfunction in these cells can lead to increased risk of miscarriage. Studies have examined NKC levels in blood and in uterine tissue in women with and without miscarriage, and results vary. Some studies show higher levels of NKC in women with RPL,[30] and other studies show no difference.[31] Some studies show higher NKC levels in the uterine tissue of RPL patients[32] while others show no difference.[33]

Proponents for testing argue that the testing is accurate and that NKC dysfunction causes miscarriages while proponents against testing argue that:[34]

1. NKC are essential for normal embryo implantation in the uterus.

NKC levels vary drastically in blood and uterine tissue, and one level does not reflect a consistent state of immune function.
3. NKC levels in the blood do not correspond to NKC levels in the uterine tissue; therefore, blood levels of NKC do not provide information on what is going on at the implantation site.
4. The laboratory tests available for NKC are inconsistent and unreliable.

Human Leukocyte Antigen (HLA) Type and Matching

HLA molecules sit on the surface of cells and help identify self and non-self cells. These molecules are coded for by a genetic complex on chromosome number 6, and each person has a unique HLA type. Dysfunction in the HLA system, the immune system's recognition process, has been proposed as a cause of RPL.

One theory is that increased sharing of HLA complexes between parents and/or between mother and baby leads to immune recognition confusion. That may seem counterintuitive since cells that recognize each other should not attack each other, but the implantation of an embryo is the acceptance of foreign genetic material, and the theory is that the system works best when the HLA molecules are highly differentiated.

Other studies investigate whether specific HLA allele prevalence is higher in patients with RPL compared to patients without RPL. In one case-control study of 588 Caucasian women with RPL and 562 Caucasian women without RPL, the HLA-DRB1*03 allele was found significantly more often in women with RPL.[35] Research is ongoing, and the significance of these findings or any intervention when found have yet to be determined.

One study about HLA typing and sex of previous live birth got a lot of attention in the press when it came out in 2008, and patients still ask about it. Nielsen et al published a study of 358 women suggesting that women with secondary RPL after the birth of a boy have a significantly lower (22%) subsequent live birth rate with they carried one of three HLA class II alleles (DRB1*15:01, -DQB1*15:01/05:02, and -DRB3*03:01) known to predispose to clinically relevant anti-HY immune reactions.[36,37] The studies are interesting, and more research is needed before broad generalizations can be determined.

In summary, experts do not agree on theories or results from studies on the impact of HLA type on risk of miscarriage and RPL. Most of the small studies in the past exploring HLA compatibility and RPL are obsolete since the laboratory tests used in the past only detected broad changes and are outdated. Hopefully, research will continue in this area, but HLA typing is not currently a typical or standard test for patients with RPL.

Cytokines

Cytokines are signaling molecules secreted from immune cells, and they usually bind to receptors on other immune cells, resulting in stimulation or suppression of an immune function. There are many different cytokines, but they are grouped into T-helper type 1 cells (Th1) and T-helper type 2 cells (Th2). The cytokines need to shift to a receptive TH2-dominant cytokine environment in pregnancy, and some argue that patients with a TH1-dominant system have a higher chance of miscarriage.[38] Some cytokines that can be tested in blood or from endometrial tissue from a uterine lining biopsy include interferon (IFN), interleukin (IL), and tumor necrosis factor (TNF). Cytokines work at close range from cell to cell, and interpretation of results from the blood or uterine tissue are likely invalid. Elevated cytokines could be a sign of immune dysfunction or could be false positive results. Some small studies have shown higher levels of certain cytokines, while others have not replicated the results, and the 2017 ESHRE RPL guidelines do not recommend testing for cytokines or cytokine polymorphisms in women with RPL.[4]

Thyroid Antibodies

These were discussed earlier in the thyroid section within this chapter and previously in Chapter 2. The presence of thyroid peroxidase antibodies (TPO), with or without other signs of thyroid disease, have been associated with an increased risk of miscarriage in some studies. Some suggest that the presence of TPO antibodies is a marker of a generalized predisposition to autoimmune dysfunction, and others suggest that patients with TPO antibodies have a decreased ability to keep up with the increased thyroid needs of pregnancy and having levothyroxine treatment established at the time of pregnancy will decrease miscarriage risk.

A well designed randomized controlled trial examining the use of levothyroxine in women with normal thyroid function but elevated TPO antibodies did NOT show decreased miscarriage rates in women.[39] In this trial, published in *JAMA* in 2017, 600 women undergoing IVF with embryo transfer with normal thyroid function and positive TPO antibodies were randomized to receive levothyroxine or a placebo, and both groups had a 10% miscarriage rate. Treating euthyroid (normally functioning thyroid) with levothyroxine did not change their rate of miscarriage. Of note – these patients were not RPL patients, and many argue that results cannot be used from a different patient population.

In summary, treatment of isolated TPO-antibody-positive RPL patients with normal functioning thyroid is controversial. Many argue that close monitoring of TSH levels while trying to conceive and in pregnancy is appropriate care.

Antinuclear Antibodies (ANA)

Also known as antinuclear factor, these are autoantibodies that bind to the nucleus in cells. There are many subtypes of ANAs, differentiated by which proteins they bind to. Elevated ANAs are associated with increased immune response in autoimmune issues, infection, and other diseases like cancer. There are many different lab assays to test for ANA, and results are inconsistent. A positive ANA result may reflect immune dysfunction, but false positives are common, and this test is rarely helpful in screening RPL patients.

Summary on Immune Testing for RPL

The recommendations from expert groups vary or are completely absent regarding immune testing for RPL. ASRM does not mention any specific immune testing in their guidelines for evaluation and treatment for RPL.[3] The Royal College of Obstetricians and Gynecologists from Britain states that evidence does not support and specifically recommends against testing for HLA incompatibility and NKC testing in blood and uterine tissue.[40] Updated ESHRE 2017 guidelines do not recommend any routine immune testing for patients with RPL.[4]

In an evidence-based summary of immune testing for RPL, Christiansen and coauthors state that testing for immune dysfunction in RPL is inherently flawed and that evidence showing a causal link between an abnormal immune test and miscarriage is weak. They caution against focusing on one specific test or group of immune cells and remind readers that there are no set guidelines for what constitutes 'abnormal' immune test results. They conclude that the immune system is complex and varied and that there is likely not one specific immune test that will consistently show an immune dysfunction in every RPL patient.[34] This does not necessarily mean there is no immune dysfunction, but it does mean the testing available to prove a dysfunctional immune system has little value.

Chapter 3.5: Immune Issues – Treatment Controversies

Immune Treatment for RPL

The immune system plays an intricate role in embryo implantation, and correcting a potential defect in this system may sound appealing to patients and physicians alike who want to decrease risks of another miscarriage in RPL. Patients can feel like their body is **broken** and rejecting a 'perfect' embryo, and the immune system is an easy target for blame. Physicians may want to give an intervention to help patients; however, testing and treatment for immune issues surrounding miscarriage is controversial. Experts agree that alterations in the immune system are essential for a successful pregnancy but do not agree on treatment options. Treatment for presumed immune dysfunction involves medications and treatments to suppress the immune system, but these treatments are not without risk.

Steroids

Steroids are used in many immune disorders to decrease inflammation and improve the symptoms associated with that inflammation, like difficulty breathing in asthma or joint pain in rheumatoid arthritis. There are many types of steroids: those naturally produced in the body and those manufactured by pharmaceutical companies to treat disease. Steroids used to treat women with RPL include corticosteroids like prednisone that suppress the immune system response and decrease inflammation, in theory to help the body accept the embryo.

One randomized controlled trial of 150 women with unexplained RPL showed higher ongoing pregnancy rates (past 20 weeks' gestation) in 74 women receiving prednisolone 5mg/day compared to 76 women receiving placebo pills.[40] Both groups in this study also received aspirin and heparin in pregnancy. One other study in which 40 unexplained RPL patients with high NKC serum levels were randomized to prednisolone treatment (20mg for six weeks then 10mg for one week then 5mg for one week) had a 60% live birth rate compared to the placebo group with 40% live birth rate.[41] Critics note small sample size and lack of power to determine significant findings in both of these studies. Professional medical groups do not recommend steroids as a treatment for RPL and warn about significant side effects with steroids, including gestational diabetes and gestational hypertension in women taking steroids in pregnancy.[3,4]

Intravenous Immunoglobulin (IVIG) Therapy

IVIG is a pooled blood product made from the collection of thousands of donations from thousands of different people donating their blood. Antibodies are isolated from the plasma portion of blood and collected into IVIG preparations. Most treatment is intravenous, but there are some subcutaneous (injected under the skin) preparations. IVIG is used to treat autoimmune diseases like Guillain-Barré syndrome and other disease states in which patients have the inability to make their own antibodies to fight infection.

Proponents for IVIG use in RPL note small studies showing benefit or anecdotal patient success stories while proponents against it argue that:
1. Large, well-designed studies show no benefit.[42,43]
2. The risks of IVIG are too high to justify using it without strong evidence to support benefit. Risks include fever, flushing, muscle pain, nausea, headache, and serious anaphylactic shock in the short term, as well as risk of long-term issues if blood products are not screened or fail to screen for communicable diseases.[44,45]

3. The cost is extremely high. Each infusion treatment can be thousands of dollars, and most treatment regimens require multiple treatments.
4. Supply is limited and should be reserved for patients with autoimmune disease and immunodeficiencies proven to benefit from use with IVIG.

Intravenous Intralipids

These are designed to provide patients who cannot use their digestive tract to digest food with calories until they can eat again. Patients who are intubated in the intensive care unit, for example, will temporarily obtain their nutrition through intravenous infusions, including lipids. Intravenous intralipids are also used to help the body clear some toxic overdoses of some anesthetic medications.

Intralipid infusions are more appealing than IVIG because they are less expensive and do not comprise a collection of blood products from thousands of people, but there is very little evidence to support using IV intralipids for RPL. One small study in 2008 showed IV intralipids lowered natural killer cell levels in the blood,[46] but we've already reviewed the lack of data showing that natural killer cells in serum impact miscarriage risk. Another clinical trial showed no benefit of IV intralipids in women with RPL.[47]

Immediate side effects can include flushing, dizziness, muscle pain, nausea and vomiting, and anaphylactic allergic reaction. Long-term side effects can include liver and kidney dysfunction and increased risk of infection and blood clots. Most infusions contain predominantly egg yolk, soybean oil, glycerine, and water, but some are high in aluminum, which can be harmful to health over time.

Anti-Tumor Necrosis Factor Alpha (anti-TNFa)

TNFa is an important part of the immune system. It's a cytokine that regulates the function of the immune system, and its dysfunction has been associated with many different diseases, from Alzheimer's disease to cancer to Crohn's disease. Anti-TNFas are a class of medications used to decrease inflammation and symptoms from the inflammation caused by overactive TNFa. Short-term risks include rashes and allergic reactions. Use of these medications have been associated with serious illnesses like the development of granulomatous diseases like tuberculosis, cancers like lymphoma and skin cancer, systemic lupus erythematosus–like syndromes, congestive heart failure, and demyelinating diseases.

Paternal Leukocyte Transfusion

This treatment (also referred to as **lymphocyte immunization therapy**) involves taking a blood sample from the male partner of a couple with RPL, isolating white blood cells (leukocytes) from his blood, and injecting his leukocytes into the female partner in an effort to build up her tolerance to his immune cells. One small, randomized trial showed a benefit for this therapy in 1985,[48] but subsequent trials and meta-analysis data have not shown a benefit.[49] This treatment is still recommended by some providers, although paternal leukocyte transfusion has been **illegal** in the US since 2002. Patients have to travel to other countries under questionable conditions for this particular immunosuppressive therapy, and randomized, therapeutic studies show no benefit of paternal leukocyte transfusion for treatment of recurrent pregnancy loss.[50] Risks include immediate allergic reactions and difficulties with the transfusion process, and long-term risks include potential harm from infections that may occur in any transfusion procedure.

Granulocyte Colony-Stimulating Factor

Granulocyte-macrophage colony-stimulating factor (GM-CSF) and granulocyte colony-stimulating factor (G-CSF) are growth factors that promote trophoblasts (embryonic cells that develop into the placenta) that have been proposed to have anti-miscarriage benefits in patients with RPL. Mechanisms remain unclear, but some animal studies have shown benefits. One randomized controlled trial published in 2009 of 68 women with unexplained RPL showed a significantly higher live birth rate in the 35 women who received subcutaneous G-CSF injections for the first trimester of pregnancy compared to 33 women who received placebo injections (82.8% live birth rate in the treatment group vs. 48.5% live birth rate in the non-treatment group).[51] Follow up studies have not shown benefits, and GM-CSF and G-CSF are not recommended for treatment for women with RPL by professional medical societies.

Summary on Immune Treatment for RPL

The recommendations from expert groups vary or are completely absent regarding immune therapy for RPL. ASRM recommends against the use of prednisone for immune suppression in RPL due to increased risk of gestational diabetes and gestational hypertension but does not address other immune therapies mentioned here.[3] The RCOG states that evidence does not support and specifically recommends against paternal cell immunization, third-party donor leukocytes, and IVIG due to increased risk of transfusion reaction, anaphylactic shock, and hepatitis.[44] RCOG also recommends against the use of anti-tumor necrosis factor agents due to risk of lymphoma and granulomatous diseases such as tuberculosis, demyelinating disease, congestive heart failure, and syndromes similar to systemic lupus erythematous.[44]

Focusing on the immune system attacking the embryo and causing RPL plays well into women's cultural tendency to feel guilty and blame themselves for miscarriages. Our society has blamed women forever for infertility, miscarriages, female and male sex of babies, and everything to do with reproduction. It's been the women's responsibility to have a baby, and if it's not happening, then she's **broken**.

With the advancements in technology and research in genetics, we've learned that sperm are responsible for the sex of babies and that most miscarriages are due to a chromosomal imbalance in the embryo. Each embryo has 23 chromosomes, half from the egg and half from the sperm; if at conception an imbalance in chromosome number occurs, the embryo can implant and develop, but at some point, the pregnancy will stop developing. This is a random occurrence, and each pregnancy is a new chance for a balanced embryo and healthy baby. It's important to note that some miscarriages have a normal chromosome balance (like a miscarriage after a genetically screened embryo in IVF). In these cases, we cannot assume that the entire genetic makeup of the embryo is normal. Each chromosome has about 25,000 genes, so even if the chromosome number is balanced, there can still be a genetic problem in the embryo that leads to miscarriage – we just cannot test for it yet.

Genetic issues in the embryo explain the women with a high number of miscarriages who go on to have a baby. These issues also explain why women with multiple miscarriages and significant poor egg quality can have babies with a donor egg; while the same woman is conceiving and carrying the pregnancy to term, she is conceiving with an embryo from a donor's egg. We have discovered genetic mutations for certain diseases like cystic fibrosis and sickle cell disease, and someday we will likely discover genetic mutations within embryos that cause miscarriage.

The adaptation of the immune system is essential for embryo implantation and a healthy pregnancy. Dysfunction in this process may lead to recurrent miscarriage, but the testing and treatment for immune dysfunction in RPL is controversial.

Proponents for immune testing and treatment cite individual studies or anecdotal evidence, meaning individual patients that had a baby with immune treatment in pregnancy after a history of RPL. Proponents against testing and treatment argue that most women with RPL will go on to have a baby without intervention. They argue that every pregnancy is a new opportunity, so a success is likely due to a new attempt, not necessarily the immune interventions. They also call attention to the potential of harm with some of the immune treatments. With any intervention, especially when the risks of treatment are high and the benefits questionable, Western medicine relies on large, well-designed studies or a systematic review of all the small studies called meta-analyses to help answer medical questions. Academic expert opinion and results from highly respected studies do not support the routine use of the immunosuppression treatment options reviewed here for unexplained RPL.

Patients with RPL are desperate for answers, and it's comforting to find an 'answer' and address an 'issue' when testing and treating immune dysfunction. We are constantly learning, and I keep an open mind for immune testing and treatment, but when the side effects and risks are high and the evidence weak, I proceed with caution in any part of my practice. I encourage patients to read, ask questions, get second opinions, and consider all alternatives before starting immunosuppressant therapy for RPL.

Chapter 3.6: Genetic Testing of Miscarriages

Cytogenetic Testing of Miscarriage

The most common cause of first trimester miscarriage is a chromosome imbalance (or **aneuploidy**) in the embryo, occurring in at least 60% of pregnancies tested.[52] The incidence of aneuploidy in miscarriages increases with age such that 80-90% of miscarriages in women conceiving in their late 30s and 40s will have aneuploidy.[53]

Testing of pregnancy tissue for chromosome imbalance is available in many clinics and hospitals. This testing involves collecting the pregnancy tissue and sending it to a lab to evaluate the chromosome number. The tissue can either be collected by D&C (dilation and curettage procedure to empty the uterus) or in some cases collected at home with a spontaneous miscarriage.

There are different types of genetic testing of pregnancy tissue. The two most commonly used techniques are conventional karyotyping and array comparative genomic hybridization. The traditional **conventional karyotyping** (metaphase karyotype testing) requires waiting for cells to develop in a lab and cannot differentiate between maternal tissue and fetal tissue. With conventional karyotyping, sometimes there is no answer because the cells failed to develop properly or there is maternal cell contamination, meaning the result is normal female (46XX), which could mean the cells were from a normal female pregnancy or that the cells tested were really from the uterine lining of the woman who conceived.

The other type of genetic testing available, **array comparative genomic hybridization,** uses a different technique to analyze chromosomes and compares the result to maternal DNA testing from a blood sample if the result is 46XX. This type of testing can rule out maternal cell contamination and give a result more often than the traditional karyotype testing. There are pros and cons to the different testing techniques.

> Many patients tell me that genetic testing was done on their miscarriages and 'everything was normal.' I always request records

> to review what test was done and whether we can really know that the pregnancy tissue had a balanced chromosome number and profile. Many times patients have a result '46XX' from metaphase karyotype testing (a traditional and common way to test miscarriages) and have been told this was normal, BUT this is wrong. This result is really a non-answer since it could be maternal cell contamination. I cannot emphasize enough how important this difference is because it changes what we know and what we don't know. This result clarifies next steps.

Proponents for this testing argue that knowing a miscarriage is due to a genetic abnormality in the embryo has psychological benefits for the patients and decreases the demand for unnecessary testing and treatment for otherwise unexplained RPL. Proponents against the testing argue that the majority of miscarriages will be abnormal anyway and that the cost does not justify the testing. Some argue that testing should only be offered in the setting of recurrent pregnancy loss but not sporadic miscarriage (meaning a first miscarriage).

I offer genetic testing of any miscarriage in my practice because it can help provide answers and clarify the next steps for a patient. For example, a couple who has a euploid (chromosomally balanced) miscarriage may not choose IVF with chromosomal screening of embryos as a next step since that intervention would not have prevented their most recent miscarriage. Each patient should have the option of testing miscarriages for genetic issues; unfortunately, this option is not discussed in the setting of diagnosis and grieving of a miscarriage. Cost of this testing is not always covered by insurance, and transparency of cost from the lab doing the test is important.

Chapter 3.7: Ovarian Reserve Testing

Ovarian Reserve Testing

Ovarian reserve testing involves blood tests and ultrasound views of the ovaries in order to understand egg quality, egg quantity, and fertility potential. We will review the testing details in more detail in Chapter 4, but for now, the controversy with this testing is whether or not it should be a part of an evaluation for RPL. No expert guidelines recommend ovarian reserve testing for a standard RPL evaluation, but proponents for testing argue that women with diminished ovarian reserve (DOR) have a higher risk of miscarriage and that knowing their fertility potential will help guide their treatment choices. Studies have shown that women with DOR have a higher percentage of embryos with chromosome imbalances[54] and a higher chance of miscarriage at younger ages due to chromosome imbalances,[55] and proponents for testing argue that DOR may explain otherwise unexplained RPL.[56]

I recommend ovarian reserve testing for my RPL patients because it helps me counsel them on the next steps moving forward.

Chapter 3.8: IVF for RPL

IVF for RPL

In vitro fertilization (IVF) with chromosomal screening of embryos is a treatment option for patients with RPL as a means for decreasing risk of miscarriage due to chromosomal imbalances in the embryos. We will review this treatment in greater detail in Chapter 4, but this option is controversial for many reasons. Proponents for this treatment option argue that the most common cause of first trimester miscarriage is a chromosomal imbalance in the embryos, and that by screening for embryos with a balanced chromosome number, the risk of miscarriage is decreased. Proponents against this treatment option argue that women's chances of a successful pregnancy conceived naturally are high without the high cost and complication of IVF, and that there is no guarantee of success with the IVF option. I have done IVF with chromosomal screening for patients with RPL in my practice but counsel each patient with regard to their own history and chances of success.

Key Points

- Research and investigation into the evaluation and treatment of miscarriage and reproduction in general are ongoing, and many options are not black and white.
- Debated testing includes inherited thrombophilia, MTHFR mutations, progesterone levels, infection screening, thyroid function, and immune testing.
- Debated treatment includes anticoagulation therapy, supplements, hormonal treatments, antibiotics, immunosuppression, and IVF with genetic screening of embryos.
- Without answers, patients are vulnerable to doing treatment that has the potential to be harmful and should consider risks to treatment before starting.

"Once you choose hope, anything's possible."
– Christopher Reeve

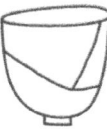

4

Genetics: The Link Between Age, Egg Quality, and Miscarriage

Genetics has opened a whole new world of understanding in human reproduction, fertility, and miscarriage over the last few decades, and we are on the verge of more discoveries every day. Through genetic testing, we have learned that most miscarriages have a chromosomal imbalance,[1] and this knowledge has opened the door to new treatment options for women with unexplained recurrent pregnancy loss (RPL). In this chapter, we will review the basics of genetics, the factors that increase the risk of miscarriage from chromosomal imbalances, and the treatment options available to decrease this risk.

Basics of Reproductive Genetics

Sit back and relax, because I'll be taking you back to high school biology for a quick review. In every cell in our body, we have 23 chromosomes (remember those 'Xs' in your textbooks?). Each chromosome holds approximately 25,000 genes linked together. Imagine a tall stack of Legos® piled up high and twisted around itself in which the genes are the Legos® and the chromosomes are the stacks of Legos® piled up like a tower. There are two copies of each chromosome in every cell in our bodies – one copy from the egg we came from and one copy from the sperm we came from. As the ryos develop and cells divide, the chromosomes replicate and divide into new cells, and information on the genes gets coded into cell functions.

If a mistake is made at fertilization between the egg and sperm, and the resulting embryo has an imbalance in chromosome number, then the resulting embryo will most likely stop developing. If the embryo has an extra chromosome (trisomy) or is missing a chromosome (monosomy), then the resulting embryo does not have a balanced set of chromosomes and will most likely result in a miscarriage. One chromosome imbalance that many people are familiar with is Down syndrome, in which a baby is born with trisomy 21 (the embryo has three copies of chromosome number 21). There are other rare chromosome imbalances that can result in live birth and there are other genetic mistakes like duplications of material, deletions of material, and more that result in miscarriage, but for the purposes of this chapter and review on genetics in miscarriage, we will focus on chromosomal imbalances that lead to first trimester miscarriage.

Why Do Mistakes Happen?

Both eggs and sperm can make mistakes when getting ready for fertilization, but the culprit is usually the egg, for reasons you'll soon understand. As eggs and sperm are developing, they should get rid of half of their chromosome copies before coming together to create a balanced embryo. Both the egg and the sperm should go through a genetic process called meiosis, in which the chromosomes are replicated and then split in half, so that the resulting egg or sperm has half of the genetic content. If an egg or sperm makes a mistake in meiosis, the resulting embryo will have a genetic imbalance, which could lead to miscarriage. Eggs and sperm develop differently, and this difference is a key link in the difference in fertility between men and women.

Get ready for more biology – this is important. Eggs are formed when women are inside their mothers' wombs, and these eggs are frozen in genetic suspension for years until ovulation. Sperm also go through meiosis, but they do this every single day – they are not suspended in genetic limbo for years like eggs. Eggs go through the first steps of meiosis in the mother's womb, but they are stopped and suspended in the process of meiosis in a stage called meiosis I. It's when the eggs ovulate (whether someone is 20 years old or 40 years old) that the genetic steps start up again, meiosis is finished, and the egg is ready to fertilize with a sperm. Sperm are made every day (millions of them), and when they are made, they are ready to go – prepped with half of the copies of chromosomes they need. Mistakes can happen with sperm, of course, but the sperm aren't sitting around for years waiting for this developmental change. Sperm are sensitive to environmental changes, but they have less time sitting around waiting to be negatively impacted. Eggs can be in limbo for years until ovulation, susceptible to impact from age and environment, and it isn't until the time of ovulation that the real genetic work must happen.

Learning this fundamental difference in male vs. female reproductive biology was like a light bulb going off for me. Finally, I could explain to patients why the fertility window is so different for men and women and why some men can conceive in their 70s (Mick Jagger!) and women cannot. It's not women's fault, it's just biology and the way we are built. No cells in our body work as well at age 40 as they do at age 20. This does not mean that all eggs are 'bad' at any given age, but it can explain why it takes longer to conceive, fertility treatment success rates are lower, and miscarriage rates increase as women age.

> I discuss genetics with patients every day. It is essential to understand why age impacts women's reproductive options more dramatically and at a younger age than men. I am an educator for my patients, and I want them to understand the why in all we do.

Egg Quality and Ovarian Reserve

My second light bulb moment as a miscarriage specialist came when I realized how many of my patients with RPL have diminished ovarian reserve or signs of poor egg quality and quantity. It all makes sense; poor egg quality means more eggs that make genetic mistakes means a higher risk of miscarriage. It's all related, connected.

Sometimes, multiple miscarriages can be a warning sign of poor egg quality. Unfortunately, there is no clear scientific consensus on what defines diminished ovarian reserve. Unlike sperm that we can examine easily outside the body, the eggs are inside the ovaries inside our bodies, and the only tests we have for egg quality are indirect. The three tests that we do have to evaluate ovarian reserve are:

1. **FSH and Estradiol** – FSH (follicle-stimulating hormone) is a gonadotropin hormone released by the pituitary gland to encourage egg maturity and development. A high FSH early in the menstrual cycle (typically tested on cycle day 3) is a warning sign of diminished ovarian reserve. I describe it to patients like the ovaries are getting tired and requiring more encouragement to do their job, meaning the pituitary gland has to pump out more FSH to get the ovary to develop a mature egg. Every lab is different, but an FSH >10mIU/mL is often considered diminished ovarian reserve.[2] The level of estradiol (a type of estrogen in the blood) needs to be checked at the same time as the FSH level to ensure that the FSH result is accurate. A high estradiol level can lower the FSH

level and make it look 'better' than it is in reality. Every lab is different, but a cycle day 3 estradiol >80pg/mL may prompt a repeat test in a subsequent menstrual cycle and can be an additional sign of diminished ovarian reserve. High estrogen levels early in a cycle can be a sign of early follicle recruitment and egg development, which can be a warning sign of diminished ovarian reserve.

2. **Anti-Müellerian Hormone (AMH)** – AMH is a blood test that can give a window into egg quantity (and maybe quality). It is a hormone made by supporting cells around eggs, and in theory, the higher the AMH level, the higher the reserve of eggs available. As a field, we are still studying AMH and figuring out what 'normal' levels are, but some experts agree that an AMH <1.0ng/mL is a sign of diminished ovarian reserve.[2] The best use of AMH is to predict the response to gonadotropin therapy in ovarian stimulation for an IVF cycle. The higher the AMH, the more eggs we can recruit in one stimulation cycle. AMH levels can help dictate IVF protocol and dose of medication and help counsel success with IVF for each patient. We should not overestimate AMH's prediction for natural fertility – very little data exists to make broad generalizations (even if the internet does so).

3. **Antral Follicle Count** – This test involves visual inspection of the ovaries with a transvaginal ultrasound and subjective counting of the number of resting follicles within the ovaries. We cannot see eggs on ultrasound (they are a single cell only seen with a high-powered microscope outside of the body), but we can see the fluid collections that surround eggs called **follicles** on ultrasound. Every menstrual cycle, women have a certain resting pool of antral follicles that are available for recruitment. Through hormone communication, usually only

one egg matures and develops to ovulate, and the others that were not selected die off. Eggs are constantly being recruited and lost, even when we're not trying to conceive or are on birth control. The higher the number of follicles seen on an ultrasound (like high AMH), the higher the reserve of eggs. Experts cannot agree on the definition of diminished ovarian reserve by antral follicle count, but in general, a total antral follicle count between both ovaries of less than six predicts poor response to some fertility treatments (also known as diminished ovarian reserve or DOR).[2]

There are other tests for ovarian reserve like inhibin B (a hormone produced in follicles that decreases with age and ovarian reserve), ovarian volume on ultrasound, and the clomiphene challenge test. These other tests are less reliable, and ASRM does not recommend routine use of these tests to determine diminished ovarian reserve.[2]

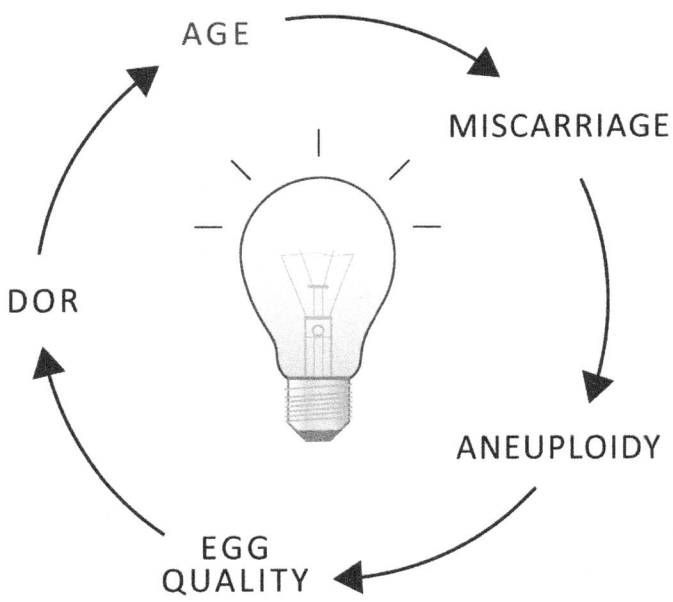

Ovarian Reserve and Miscarriage

So how does this all tie together with miscarriage? Age, diminished ovarian reserve, fertility, miscarriage, genetics – it's all intertwined, so let's review some findings that help tie it all together:

- Fertility decreases with age.[3]
- Risk of miscarriage increases with age such that a woman's chance of miscarriage at an age less than 35 years old is 9-12%, but at age 40 years, the risk of miscarriage is 50%.[4]
- Studies examining IVF in women with advancing reproductive age show a higher percentage of aneuploid (chromosomally unbalanced) embryos[5] and higher risk of miscarriage[6] with age.
- Women with diminished ovarian reserve have a higher percentage of aneuploid embryos[7] and a higher risk of miscarriage.[8]
- The most common cause of first trimester miscarriage is aneuploidy in the embryo.[4]
- The risk of aneuploidy in miscarriages increases with a woman's age.[9]
- Women with DOR and RPL have a higher percentage of aneuploid embryos, despite their age.[8]
- People with recurrent miscarriage have a higher incidence of diminished ovarian reserve at a younger age than people without recurrent miscarriage.[10]

Diminished ovarian reserve is not traditionally associated with recurrent miscarriage, and no professional medical societies at the time of this publication recommend testing ovarian reserve in patients with RPL, but I have done this in my own practice for over 10 years. I use it for counseling patients about their goals and outcomes with all treatment options. I discuss IVF with genetic screening of embryos with patients, and some RPL patients choose this option for many reasons. In my practice, I have observed two patterns: a high number of my patients had DOR at a young age, and patients with RPL seem to have a higher percentage of aneuploid embryos with IVF at a younger age. I formally studied these trends and published my findings in peer-reviewed journals.

In the first study, 239 patients with unexplained RPL did IVF with genetic screening of embryos, and 102 patients had at least one euploid blast to transfer.[8] The outcomes were analyzed by patients' ovarian reserve status, and DOR was defined as FSH>10 IU/mL and/or AMH<1.0ng/mL. Patients with DOR had a higher percentage of aneuploid blastocysts (57% vs 49%, P=0.03) and a higher incidence of no euploid embryos to transfer (25% vs 13%, P=0.02). The higher rate of aneuploidy in blastocysts was most significant in patients aged <38 years (67% vs 53%, P=0.04). Implantation rates after transfer of euploid blastocysts were similar in the two groups (61% compared with 59%, P=0.4), and miscarriage rates were low (14% and 10%, P=0.08). I observed that unexplained RPL patients with DOR have a higher percentage of aneuploid blastocysts and risk of no euploid embryo to transfer compared with unexplained RPL patients with normal ovarian reserve testing. The difference is most significant in patients aged <38 years. It is reassuring that if a euploid embryo was found with IVF and transferred, patients with RPL and DOR have similar outcomes compared with patients with RPL and normal ovarian reserve testing. It is also important to counsel patients before IVF that there is a chance no euploid blasts will be found to transfer and that risk increases with DOR.

I wanted to learn more about the group of RPL patients less than 38 years old who had a higher rate of aneuploid embryos than expected for their age. I reviewed data from patients seeking care in our clinic for RPL and compared incidence of DOR by age and cause of RPL.[10] In the 264 patients with recurrent pregnancy loss included,

87 had an identifiable cause and 177 patients had no cause of RPL identified (unexplained RPL). A higher percentage of patients with unexplained RPL had DOR compared to patients with a known cause for RPL (48% vs 29%, p = .005). This finding was most significant in patients less than 38 years old compared to patients 38 years old and older (22% vs. 12%, p = .04). In my own practice, I am observing a higher rate of DOR in younger patients with RPL, and I wonder if DOR can be an explanation for RPL in some patients. Although current professional guidelines do not include ovarian reserve testing as a part of routine evaluation for RPL, I find it helpful in counseling patients through all options moving forward.

Risk of miscarriage increases with age of eggs and DOR. Most experts agree that women are born with a finite number of eggs and that many of the eggs available for ovulation near menopause are of poor quality. Recurrent miscarriage can be a warning sign of diminished ovarian reserve and a potentially decreased fertility potential, but not everyone with DOR will have miscarriages, and not everyone with recurrent miscarriages will have DOR. The relationship between age, DOR, and miscarriage has shed light on why some women may be at a higher risk of miscarriage than others and helped shift focus away from fear and the unknown to focus more on the issues at hand and what can be done about them. This link between diminished ovarian reserve and miscarriage is not a predictor of outcomes for everyone.

> Important reminder: All it takes is a good egg and a good sperm and all the stars aligning to have a successful pregnancy. Every pregnancy is a new opportunity.

The knowledge regarding genetics in reproduction has led to two paths in treatment for patients with unexplained RPL – one path focuses on genetic screening of embryos before implantation via IVF and the other path focuses on maximizing health before conception to improve genetic function of eggs and sperm. These paths do not have to be mutually exclusive.

IVF as a Treatment for RPL

Genetic testing of embryos has been in practice for over 20 years. This process involves biopsying a cell or cells away from a developing embryo and testing that cell for genetic content that should represent the rest of the embryo. The technology has developed dramatically over the last 20 years, along with other leaps and bounds in assisted reproductive technology. We can now test several cells from a day 5 or 6 embryo (called a blastocyst) instead of a single cell from a day 3 embryo and increase accuracy of testing. The two most common types of genetic testing of embryos are PGT-M and PGT-A.

- **PGT-M** – Preimplantation genetic testing for monogenic/single gene disorders, in which we are testing for specific genetic mutations for hundreds of different genetic diseases. Examples include testing for mutations that lead to cystic fibrosis, sickle cell disease, and hundreds more. Terminology changes frequently, and this used to be called PGD or preimplantation diagnosis.

- **PGT-A** – Preimplantation genetic testing for aneuploidy, in which we test for all 23 chromosome pairs. Chromosome imbalances like trisomy (extra chromosome) and monosomy (missing a chromosome) in an embryo can be a common cause of first trimester miscarriage. This is the most common type of genetic testing done on embryos and has changed terminology many times. It can still be called preimplantation genetic screening (PGS), comprehensive chromosomal screening (CCS), or chromosomal screening (CS).

❑ **PGT-SR** – Preimplantation genetic testing for chromosome structural rearrangements is the type of testing used on embryos when screening for balanced translocations and inversions. In approximately 3% of couples with RPL, one of the partners will have a balanced translocation that increases the risk of miscarriage – see Chapter 2 for a detailed review of the role of balanced translocations in miscarriage.

Advances in genetic testing technology have led providers to use genetic screening of embryos for many types of patients, including RPL patients who do not need IVF to conceive but are doing it in hopes of selecting euploid (chromosomally balanced embryos) for transfer to decrease risk of another miscarriage.

Before we start an evaluation for RPL, I warn patients that we most likely will not find an answer as to why they are miscarrying because, while the testing focuses on issues we can discover in the people who are conceiving, the most common cause of miscarriage is a genetic issue in the embryo(s). We review options for treatment before and during the next pregnancy that can optimize their chances of success. If we assume that the most common cause of miscarriage is a chromosomal imbalance within the embryo that is unique to each miscarriage, then the options are either to continue to try to conceive naturally (expectant management) or to actively screen embryos for chromosomal imbalances before implantation, which requires in vitro fertilization (IVF) and genetic screening of the embryos. This is quite an extreme choice, trying naturally vs. IVF, and there is no 'right answer' for all patients. I review IVF with patients because it is considered a treatment option for unexplained RPL, but by no means is it the right fit for everyone. Before I review IVF, I remind patients that without any testing or intervention on my part, most women with RPL will go on to have a baby in the next five years.[11]

Controversy: IVF for RPL

Experts are divided on whether IVF with genetic screening of embryos should be a treatment option for patients with RPL. Proponents of this practice argue that women will decrease their risk of another miscarriage, and proponents against it argue that women have a high chance of successful pregnancy without this high cost and complicated intervention that doesn't even have a guarantee of success. Some studies have shown that IVF with genetic screening of embryos will decrease women's risk of miscarriage compared to their own risk based on age and miscarriage history.[12] Other studies have shown that IVF with genetic screening does not necessarily decrease time to successful pregnancy[13] and may not be cost effective.[14]

I counsel women about all options and keep an open mind while they are on their journey. If IVF with genetic testing were free, easy, and a 100% guarantee of a baby, then it would likely be appealing to most patients, but this is unfortunately not the case. IVF has its limitations, and success is only as good as the eggs and sperm we have to work with.

The tabloids with their 'mommy glorification' of celebrities make it seem like as long as you are rich and famous enough, you can have a baby with IVF, but this is not the case. The media also sensationalizes mothers at advanced reproductive age. When Janet Jackson announced that she was canceling her world tour to focus on family in 2016 and subsequently announced that she was expecting a baby at age 50, the tabloids went crazy about how amazing it was. I agreed that it was a wonderful announcement, but I wrote a blog for *Buzzfeed* reflecting on what a missed learning opportunity it was.[15] Janet Jackson is absolutely entitled to her privacy, but without also reporting on the limitations of egg freezing and the high use of donor eggs in women conceiving after age 42, this announcement left most women who haven't achieved the family they desired feeling inadequate and asking, 'Why not me?'

I was impressed with *People* magazine's 2018 article, "Everything You Need to Know About Getting Pregnant in Your 40s, as More Stars Have Babies Near 50." After listing Brigitte Nielsen expecting a baby at 54, Rachel Weisz delivering at age 48, and Halle Berry delivering at age 47, they interview Dr. Zev Williams, reproductive endocrinologist from Columbia University in New York, who states that the chance of conceiving naturally after age 42 is less than 1%. The article even reviews the limitations of the age of the eggs and options like egg freezing, donor egg, and embryo donation!

Patients in my practice who choose to proceed with IVF and genetic screening of embryos for RPL are usually age 35 or older, have had a previous miscarriage tested and shown to be aneuploid, have the financial burden of IVF eased, typically with insurance coverage, or are so emotionally drained that they cannot consider facing another pregnancy without some intervention to decrease the risk of another miscarriage. The choice is very personal, and I reassure women who choose not to do IVF or who cannot do so for any reason that IVF for RPL is not a magic answer. There are women who miscarry with a tested embryo and there are women who go on to have babies without IVF.

IVF as a Fertility Preservation Option

While I review all options, I do discuss IVF as a fertility preservation option, especially when patients are starting their families later in life. Embryos can be cryopreserved now and used later with great success. We have decades of experience with embryo freezing in fertility treatment, and this is a wonderful option for many patients. If someone's ideal family is two or more children and they are starting their family at an advanced age, we review the long-term plan. If someone conceives at age 40, they are pregnant for about a year and do not usually start trying until a year after they deliver. And trying for a baby at age 42 is significantly more difficult than at age 40. The process of patients using IVF to cryopreserve multiple euploid embryos (more than one embryo that has been screened for balanced chromosome number) before attempting conception is usually called **embryo banking**. It's a form of fertility preservation because it's maximizing someone's present fertility in the hopes of keeping options open in the future.

Some of the most difficult and heartfelt conversations I have with patients are those who want to do IVF but have significant diminished ovarian reserve (DOR). For these women, IVF is less successful no matter what technology we have. I explain to them that IVF is not magic, meaning it does not create eggs, but IVF is science, meaning if eggs are there to recruit, then we can recruit them in an IVF cycle.

In a natural cycle, the pituitary gland makes enough gonadotropins (hormones like follicle-stimulating hormone, or FSH) to recruit one egg to ovulate, and the others that were available (antral follicles) die off. IVF takes advantage of these other potential recruits by giving the body a higher dose of gonadotropins (those daily shots people talk about in their IVF cycle) to nourish these others along to maturity as well and ultimately retrieve them out of the body at 'ovulation.'

> IVF is like an amplified menstrual cycle – recruiting and retrieving eggs that would have been lost in that cycle anyway.

If someone has a good reserve of eggs, we can recruit a good number of eggs in IVF. It's a numbers game and also about statistics – the more eggs, the more embryos, the higher chance we'll have embryos that screen for a balanced set of chromosomes. The fewer the eggs, the lower the chances we'll find an embryo that has the potential to become a baby.

Women with diminished ovarian reserve can consider IVF with genetic screening of embryos but need to understand the hurdles involved and the potential need for multiple IVF stimulation cycles to find euploid embryos. In some cases, when women have significantly poor ovarian reserve test results, I counsel them that they may have a similar chance of success continuing to try naturally compared to IVF, which baffles them. IVF is viewed by the public as the penultimate fertility treatment. And while it is absolutely amazing what we can do with it today, its biggest limitation is egg quantity and quality. I'm waiting for science to:

1. Find a way to predict which menstrual cycle is ideal for doing IVF to find a good egg.
2. Change eggs to act younger and go through genetic changes at ovulation correctly.
3. Find a way to stop eggs from constantly being lost through our reproductive years.

Until then, we work with what we have and keep trying, regrouping, reviewing options, and moving forward.

IVF With Donor Egg

When talking about the limitations of IVF in women with DOR, we talk about alternative family-building options like adoption and donor eggs. If the egg quality or egg supply is depleted, patients can still conceive, carry a child, and complete their family with a donor egg. If a limitation for success with IVF is the egg and someone has significant DOR, we cannot change that, but that person can still carry a baby to term with a donated egg or embryo.

The success rates for donor eggs are that of the age of the eggs the patients are using. This really surprises people, but the younger the eggs are, the higher the chance they can go through the genetic changes required at ovulation successfully and result in a balanced embryo. The urgency to conceive and beat the biological clock is so ingrained in women that I try to get them to relax a little once they are considering using a donor egg. They are anxious to start their family, of course, but their success rate with a donor egg is the same today as a year from today, so they can take a breath, consider whether they want to continue to try naturally, and take the time they need to learn more about the donor egg option and whether it's the right choice for them.

> Many women have a hard time grasping the concept that their eggs could be the cause of recurrent pregnancy loss because they have been so convinced it was their body that rejected a perfectly "normal" embryo. IVF can be used as an embryo selection tool (selecting for embryos that form from genetically balanced eggs and sperm), but it cannot improve the quality of the eggs and sperm. When a woman has significantly diminished ovarian reserve and/or advanced reproductive age, egg donation can be a good option to consider.

What Are the Other Options?

After I teach patients about the intimate relationship between egg quality, genetics, and miscarriage, whether patients are planning IVF or continuing to try naturally, they often ask, 'Is there anything I can do to make my eggs better?' There are theories, studies, blogs, websites, books, and loads of resources claiming that certain diets, supplements, and lifestyle changes will improve egg quality. Patients and providers alike are looking for the 'youth serum' for eggs – the medication, treatment, food, or supplement that will make eggs act younger and do their genetic work at ovulation correctly. Fads come and go, but I counsel patients on healthy lifestyle modifications, and I'll review some of the most important of these in the next chapter.

Key Points
- The most common cause of miscarriage is a chromosomal imbalance in the embryo.
- Risk of miscarriage increases with advanced reproductive age.
- Women with diminished ovarian reserve have a higher risk of miscarriage.
- Women with RPL can have a higher risk of diminished ovarian reserve.
- A link between age, egg quality, diminished ovarian reserve, and miscarriage can be genetics.
- IVF with genetic screening of embryos can be a treatment option for women with recurrent miscarriage, but it is not the only option, and it has its limitations.

> "Look deep into nature, and then you will understand everything better."
> – Albert Einstein

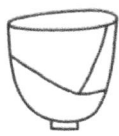

5

Lifestyle Modifications: Optimize Health and Decrease Miscarriage Risk

Regardless of the treatments and interventions, I recommend that every person trying to conceive try to maximize their health. Problems with fertility and recurrent miscarriage may be a window into overall well-being, and we can take it as motivation to improve our wellness. I approach this counseling carefully with patients because I do not want them leaving my office feeling guilty about past poor habits, and I do not want them to develop new habits that may be even worse.

I say two things to patients every day:
1. "Everything in moderation, even moderation." I can't remember where I heard or read this, but it resonated with me.
2. "Perfection is 80%." I read this Chinese proverb in *Making Babies*, a book on fertility by Jill Blakeway and Sami David.[1]

Both sayings emphasize prioritizing health and well-being, but within reason. We cannot eliminate everything we enjoy in our efforts to become parents, and we cannot make ourselves martyrs on our family-building journey. The more we lose joy, the higher the chance we lose ourselves in the process.

In this chapter, we'll review the lifestyle modifications that may impact overall health and well-being, including weight, tobacco, alcohol, marijuana, caffeine, environmental toxins, exercise, and sleep. We'll review the research available regarding impact on risk of miscarriage and recurrent pregnancy loss, and I'll add my own typical counseling guidelines to help with common questions. There is no one single recommendation that fits every person, so, as with every guideline outlined in this book, please review your care with your physician.

Chapter 5.1: Lifestyle Modifications

Maintain a Healthy Weight

Being either underweight or overweight can increase risk of miscarriage or other poor obstetric outcomes.[2,3] Body mass index (BMI) is a common measure of a 'healthy weight,' and guidelines recommend a BMI between 19-25 as ideal for conception. BMI classifications in medicine are as follows: 25-$29.9 kg/m^2$ is considered overweight, 30-$34.9 kg/m^2$ is considered obese, and a BMI over $40 kg/m^2$ is considered morbidly obese. One study showed that the risk of sporadic and recurrent miscarriage was significantly higher in women with a BMI >$30 kg/m2$.[4] Go online to find a simple BMI calculator and plug in your height and weight for a rough estimate of where you are.

Please note that BMI is an easy universal measure to help research studies compare data, but it does NOT give the full picture of health. BMI cut offs and definitions are medical guidelines used in research to investigate the impact of weight on health issues, but weight can be a very personal topic, and people can be healthy at a high BMI. We cannot put patients into boxes based on numbers on a scale, but we can review issues, answer questions, and offer support. Weight can be an extremely emotional topic for people, and many patients report negative interactions with medical providers in the past. A discussion on weight and reproductive health can focus on education and counseling but should never end in shame or guilt.

I approach this topic delicately and encourage patients to improve their nutrition and exercise routines with the goal of being their healthiest self. I warn people away from focusing too much on a number on a scale, because a myopic view can lead to unhealthy habits and discouragement when goals aren't met. Someone can calorie restrict or over-exercise and lose pounds but end up making their reproductive health worse. A key is identifying changeable habits that result in long-term success. The results take time and patience, but lasting change needs just that.

> Optimizing weight is not a quick fix. It can take years to build habits that leave someone consistently under or overweight, and it will take time to reflect and build new habits for lasting change.

Ideas for Optimizing Weight
1. Find a registered dietitian, nutritionist, or physical trainer to help review current habits and kickstart a new routine.
2. Find a positive, encouraging weight loss buddy (in person or online) – accountability is a great motivator.
3. Get an interactive activity monitor you can wear on your wrist or use with your smartphone to keep track of your progress.
4. Use an activity journal or nutrition app on your phone.
5. Try new habits you can stick with, like walking 30 minutes multiple times a week, cutting out sugary soda and juices, and getting a minimum of seven hours of sleep each night.
6. Get creative and be patient with yourself and your body.
7. Stay kind and patient with yourself – making your health a priority is the first step.

Tobacco Use

Cigarette smoking in both partners as well as secondhand smoke exposure in pregnancy have been associated with increased risk of poor pregnancy outcomes. Maternal cigarette smoking has been shown to decrease the function of the placenta and increase the risk of miscarriage, preterm birth, low birth weight, and still birth.[5] Paternal smoking has also been associated with an increased risk of miscarriage regardless of maternal smoking status in one prospective study of 526 couples.[6] Secondhand smoke from living with a smoker has also been associated with increased risk of miscarriage.[7]

Other forms of nicotine (like e-cigarettes and vaping) and other forms of tobacco (like cigars and chewing tobacco) have not been specifically studied in relationship to miscarriage, but I recommend stopping any form of tobacco exposure and only using nicotine substitutes as a temporary means to quit using tobacco or nicotine permanently.

Limit Caffeine

Increased caffeine consumption has been associated with increased risk of miscarriage, but studies differ in what they quantify as too much caffeine. Observational studies have shown a dose-dependent association between caffeine intake and miscarriage.[8] One study found that both women and men who had more than two servings of caffeinated beverages per day had an increased risk of miscarriage.[9] One retrospective case control study suggested that higher caffeine intake was a risk factor for RPL since women with over 300mg of caffeine per day had a 3x higher likelihood of RPL compared to women who consumed <150mg of caffeine most days.[10]

> **How much caffeine is in your...**
> - Cup of drip coffee: 95-200mg per 8oz
> - Espresso drink: 40-75mg per 1oz
> - Caffeinated tea: 25-30mg per 8oz
> - Soft drink/soda: 30-50mg per 12oz
> - Energy drink: 100-200mg per 12oz
>
> (Amount depends on brand, size of drink, etc.)

I live in Seattle, WA (home of Starbucks and a huge coffee culture), and my telling people to quit coffee can be like taking away a lifeline for some people. Remember: "Everything in moderation." Without knowing exactly how much is too much, I tell patients that no caffeine is the most conservative choice, but a single small cup of coffee in the morning is likely okay.

Breaking the habit of multiple cups of coffee a day can be made easier with a transition plan. Try gradually switching to decaffeinated coffee (use water-pressed, not chemically decaffeinated coffee to avoid harmful toxins), then to a green tea that has low caffeine content, then to a non-caffeinated tea. You may find that it's the routine of preparing a hot beverage and enjoying it that you crave, not the actual caffeine. Try it!

> Don't assume decaffeinated coffee is a better option. Many companies use toxic solvents like methylene chloride to process caffeine out of coffee beans before roasting. If you choose decaffeinated coffee, research and invest in a company that uses a water-based technique for decaffeination.

Limit Alcohol and Stop Use When Pregnant

Drinking alcohol during pregnancy is well known for causing fetal alcohol syndrome, a collection of physical and mental disabilities in children. But drinking alcohol in early pregnancy may also be associated with increased risk of miscarriage.[11] One case control study showed a dose-dependent increased risk of miscarriage with alcohol consumption in any level of regular alcohol intake.[12] Women with 14 or more alcoholic drinks per week had the highest risk of miscarriage, but even regular once a week alcohol intake showed increased risk. Some research shows an association between paternal alcohol consumption and increased risk of miscarriage.[13]

I tell my fertility patients and miscarriage patients to limit alcohol while trying to conceive and stop altogether with a positive pregnancy test. By limiting alcohol, I mean limit to special occasions and celebrations. Everyday alcohol use is common in many cultures; many people associate a glass of wine or a beer at the end of the day with relaxing and winding down for the evening. Alcohol can be a reward to end a tough day, but it can become a toxic habit. It takes a lot of work for your liver and kidneys to flush out toxins in alcohol – not just the alcohol itself, but all the preservatives and coloring that go into many alcoholic drinks.

Alcohol is a sedative and relaxing at first, so it puts you to sleep, but it disrupts REM sleep (our deep sleep) later in the night as your body metabolizes it. Alcohol also suppresses breathing and worsens snoring, which disrupts sleep. These effects can be seen with one to two drinks but can worsen with heavier drinking. Even if you do not wake up, you are not sleeping as well and you'll feel less rested the following day with alcohol in your system. Try eliminating alcohol for a few weeks and note any changes in your energy level and productivity.

> If alcohol has become a habit to help with the transition from your work day to a relaxing evening, one trick to help change is switching to a different nightly drink like sparkling water. You may find it's the transition routine that you crave – not the actual alcohol.

Avoid Marijuana and Other Drugs

With legalization of marijuana in some states (including Washington State, where I practice), it seems like more patients are using it (or just more comfortable telling me as their doctor). Patients can be surprised when I recommend stopping it because there is a feeling by some that it is 'natural' and 'healthy' and should not impact overall health.

Studies examining marijuana use and risk of miscarriage are limited, and to date, no studies have shown an increased risk of miscarriage in mothers using marijuana.[14] However, studies have shown a detrimental effect of marijuana on both female[15] and male fertility,[16] and I recommend all my patients, both those trying to conceive and those who are pregnant, to avoid marijuana.

We tend to assume marijuana is safe and 'natural' because it is plant-based; however, if you are not growing and processing the marijuana yourself, you cannot be sure what toxins may be present; and even if you are, there is no certainty that any exposure is safe when trying to conceive or while pregnant. It's better to be safe until we know more.

Cocaine and other drugs have also been associated with increased risk of miscarriage[17] and poor pregnancy outcomes and should be avoided.

Modify Exercise

Patients often ask about exercise routines and risk to pregnancy. Some women are so worried about doing anything to risk a miscarriage that they stop working out completely. Others fall into a pattern of intense exercise in the first half of their menstrual cycle and then minimal or absent exercise after ovulation once they have the potential of being pregnant. Excessive exercise has been associated with fertility issues, but guidelines and experts do not agree on recommendations for exercise routines that decrease risk of miscarriage.[18] A review article examining all available evidence concluded 'more studies are warranted,' meaning there is no conclusive data yet.[19]

I tell patients that exercise is important and recommend that they do some type of exercise on a regular basis – something they can do throughout the menstrual cycle and pregnancy. I do not recommend intense training for a marathon or the popular high-intensity exercises that are available like boot camps, but this is my opinion based on available data. With intense exercise, our bodies create the stress hormone cortisol and shift energy away from digestion and reproduction to survival mode. With intense exercise, blood flow shifts away from reproductive organs to more vital organs like the heart and brain. I recommend low-intensity exercise like walking, light weights, jogging, yoga, and Pilates. Focus on restorative exercise and movement, not high-intensity sessions with bursts of energy.

Make Sleep a Priority

No definitive studies have directly linked poor sleep with increased risk of miscarriage, but sleep is an essential part of our overall health and well-being. Disturbances in sleep such as too little sleep or sleep-disordered breathing like sleep apnea can lead to disturbances in hormonal and cardiovascular health. Sleep disturbances can result in menstrual cycle irregularity, prolactin disorders, and fertility issues, and one study suggests that there could be a link between obstructive sleep apnea and miscarriages.[20] I cannot emphasize enough the importance of sleep for mental and physical well-being.

Sleep tips and goals:
1. You need a minimum of seven to eight hours of sleep each night, so plan ahead: if you know you need to wake up at 6:00 am, then be in bed by 10:00 pm.
2. Routine is key for sleep – try to stick to similar hours of getting to bed and waking up every day – weekdays and weekends.
3. Avoid caffeine in the afternoon or evening.
4. Avoid alcohol since it is a sleep disruptor (see the section on alcohol above).
5. Make your bedroom cool, dark, and quiet.
6. Prep for sleep:
    - ❏ Avoid screens (phone, TV, laptop) at least one hour before bed.
    - ❏ Avoid exercise one to two hours before bed.
    - ❏ Calm down with a book, journal writing, meditation, or a warm bath.
    - ❏ Find a pre-bedtime routine that works for you and stick with it as best you can.

Chapter 5.2: Environmental Exposures and Miscarriage

Patients ask me every day about environmental toxins and reproductive health. We live in a modern world of conveniences and technology, and with that comes exposures to chemicals, plastics, and many substances that may impact our health. I counsel with caution about the impact of environmental toxins because I have seen patients become obsessed with limiting exposures to a point that can be debilitating. Remember, "Everything in moderation." We should be aware of substances and limit exposures but not go so far overboard that it becomes an obsession. I will review the evidence around environmental toxins and reproductive health and end with an approachable checklist for you to consider.

DDT (Pesticide)

DDT (or 1,1,1-trichloro–2,2'bis(p-chlorophenyl) ethane) was developed in 1874, used in World War II to decrease the spread of malaria, and adopted commercially in the United States as a pesticide for crops in the 1940s. DDT is an estrogen and androgen receptor modulator, meaning it directly impacts female and male hormonal functions. Its environmental impact can be seen in declining bird populations and birth defects in small mammals,[21] and ultimately, its association with miscarriage and other poor obstetric outcomes in humans led to its ban in developing countries in the 1970s.[22] Even though DDT is banned for use in the US today, we may still be exposed. DDT may be on imported food since many countries still use it as a pesticide. And DDT's chemical stability allows it to persist in nature all along the food chain (animals eating crops treated with DDT) for decades, so that we may still be exposed from use in the US from years ago. Other pesticides have not been studied as extensively as DDT, but I recommend trying to eat organic, local produce and meat whenever possible and washing fruits and vegetables thoroughly before eating.

BPA (Bisphenol A)

BPA (2,2-bis(4-hydroxyphenyl) propane) was first synthesized in 1891 as a synthetic estrogen for the pharmaceutical industry. Since its discovery as a powerful epoxy resin and use in polycarbonate plastics in the 1950s, production and use of this chemical has grown exponentially in the making of many household products like plastic water bottles, baby bottles, food packaging like the lining of canned food and take out containers, receipts from cash registers, and more. It is now one of the highest-volume chemicals produced worldwide.

BPA as an estrogenic compound has been linked to many reproductive disorders such as polycystic ovarian syndrome, infertility, endometriosis, and thyroid disease.[23] It has been found in follicular fluid surrounding developing eggs, endometrial tissue within the uterus, and in high levels in the urine of women with miscarriages.[24] Some studies suggest the endocrine disruption of BPA may affect embryo implantation,[25] and other studies find that BPA may affect chromosomal function within eggs, leading to miscarriage.[26]

In 2012, the United States Food and Drug Administration (FDA) banned BPA use in baby bottles. BPA use in everyday items and especially items containing food remains controversial, with research and some experts calling for more bans and national and international expert groups and panels saying BPA is not a health concern and should not be banned. Until research can show it's safe, I recommend limited exposure to plastics. BPA is the most studied and reported on chemical in plastics, and buying "BPA free" plastic doesn't mean you are not being exposed to other harmful chemicals, so consider switching as much plastic as you can to glass or stainless steel since there are many different chemicals in plastic.

Ways to limit BPA exposure:
- ❏ Switch to a stainless steel or glass water bottle.
- ❏ Limit canned food – switch to fresh or frozen options.
- ❏ Eat more whole foods – less processed means less packaging.
- ❏ Switch from storing food and leftovers in plastic containers to glass or stainless steel options.
- ❏ Avoid heating plastics that touch food since heat allows the BPA and other potential toxins to leach from plastic containers straight into your food:

- ❏ Switch food from microwavable plastic containers to glass or ceramic before heating.
- ❏ Do not put plastic in the dishwasher – hand wash it.
- ❏ Think about your coffee or tea makers – the popular pod system for making these warm beverages uses plastics to store the coffee or tea, and boiling water is pouring through the plastic right into your cup. Automatic coffee makers usually send hot water through plastics as well. Switch to a French press or pour-over system with glass for hot beverages and make tea the old-fashioned way with a kettle.
- ❏ BPA is in many thermal paper products. Avoid handling paper receipts and other thermal paper (like airline and concert tickets) whenever possible. Fortunately, we live in the digital age and can have some receipts and tickets emailed to us instead of printed out.

> Don't fall for the marketing gimmick 'BPA-free' since bisphenol A is only one of many bisphenols. A plastic may be free of BPA, but it can be full of other bisphenols, phthalates, and other endocrine disruptors that can harm reproductive and overall health.

Phthalates

Phthalates or phthalate esters are chemicals used since the 1920s to soften plastics and are found in a wide variety of products in multiple industries. They are found in PVC pipes and other building materials, gel coating for medications and supplements, IV tubing, and many medical supplies. Phthalates are used to stabilize fragrances in many home and personal care products like shampoo, lotion, cosmetics, perfume, and scented candles. Approximately eight million tons of plasticizers are consumed globally every year, and the Centers for Disease Control found metabolites for phthalates in the urine of over 90% of Americans with a random sampling.[27]

Phthalates have been associated with developmental abnormalities of the male reproductive system, miscarriage, endometriosis, and low sperm counts.[28] Phthalates have both progesterone and aromatase activity and disrupt the reproductive system on many levels.[29] Studies in mice have shown that as the exposure to phthalates increases, issues with ovulation, estrogen effects, and disrupted gene expression increase as well.[30] Studies in humans show higher rates of phthalate exposure are associated with lower rates of mature eggs in IVF,[29] lower embryo implantation rates,[30] and higher miscarriage rates.[31]

Ways to limit phthalate exposure:
- ❏ Phthalates are found in plastics, so follow the same tips for limiting plastic exposure to food and heat listed in the BPA recommendations above.
- ❏ Decrease meat and dairy consumption – these foods are an excellent source of protein and other nutrients like calcium, but plastics are used extensively in the meat and dairy industry to process the products. The phthalate exposure through processing gets passed on to you when you eat.
- ❏ Most scents in household products are stabilized with phthalates:
  - ❏ Skip scented air fresheners and sprays and try baking soda in trash cans and the fridge to absorb odors.
  - ❏ Avoid heavily fragranced candles, laundry detergent, etc. – try fragrance-free products and use carefully screened essential oils if you enjoy scents.
  - ❏ Avoid scented household cleaning products and try a mix of vinegar and water instead, or at least switch to the less toxic cleaning products that are now more widely available.
  - ❏ Check your personal care products:

- ❏ Choose fragrance free options.
- ❏ Avoid perfumes.

> 'Fragrance' listed as an ingredient in a product can be a warning sign of toxins. A product's smell or fragrance can be considered a trade secret, and companies can omit listed ingredients that are used to create or maintain smell in a product. Phthalates can stabilize smell in a product, so they may be omitted from a list of ingredients in some cases.

Personal Care Products/The Beauty Industry

The beauty industry is not well regulated in the United States. Only 11 ingredients have been banned for use in personal care products in the United States compared to over 600 in Canada and over 1,300 in Europe. Since the last law to limit chemicals in cosmetics in the US passed in 1938, an estimated 80,000 have been developed for use in household products but not tested on humans for toxicity. The attitude in the US is to assume safety until proven otherwise, and companies claim that the amount of endocrine disruptors in their products are too small to cause harm. Well, other countries have lower thresholds, and no one seems to be taking into account how many different products we use daily and the additive impact of the chemicals in all the different products. Take a day and count the number of products you use: soap, shampoo, conditioner, shaving cream, toothpaste, mouthwash, lotion, foundation, mascara, concealer, lipstick, laundry detergent on clothing, keep going. We cannot eliminate our exposure to toxins, but smart choices with the products we use daily can decrease our overall exposure.

Three ways to find cleaner products
1. Read each label yourself and look up each ingredient – remember, 'fragrance' as an ingredient can be a code word for

phthalates and other toxic ingredients if considered a trade secret by the company producing the product (see the section on phthalates above).
2. Look up your products in a database like the Environmental Working Group (ewg.org) or Think Dirty® – but realize that not every product is listed, each database has different criteria, and that some of these databases require clean companies to pay to be listed, which leads to bias.
3. Find companies that make clean products:
   a. Beautycounter® is a beauty company not only making cleaner products but also lobbying for more transparency in the beauty industry.
   b. Some companies like Follain or Credo Beauty vet products for you and provide a database to choose from.

You have to do the work to find safer products. You cannot rely on FDA oversight or meaningless marketing terminology like 'natural.' It's easy to get overwhelmed if this is the first time you're learning about toxins in products. Don't let that happen – realize that small changes make a big difference and make changes at your own pace.

> I tell my patients to take it one product at a time. When it's time to replace a product like your favorite shampoo, research the product and see if there is a toxin-free option available.

Chapter 5.3: Practice Self-Care

We've discussed a lot of specific lifestyle modifications so far: weight, exercise, substances, and toxins. Something I emphasize for my patients (and myself) is self-care. You must make yourself a priority while on your family-building journey. It's very easy to put others' needs first – whether it be the needs of your partner, your boss, your family, or your friends – but you need to take care of yourself. It's okay to make yourself your focus for now, and you'll be a better partner and friend, and more productive at work, if you are taking care of yourself. Miscarriage takes a huge physical and emotional toll. There will be time in the future to do all the things you want to or feel you should, but for now, make yourself your priority.

Tips for self-care:
- Be patient and kind with yourself. Don't criticize yourself or beat yourself up about the things you could have done differently. Just allow yourself the space and time you need to grieve and heal while you learn how to implement positive changes in your health and life.
- Make sleep a priority (I cannot emphasize this enough). Your mind and body need sleep to restore, heal, and function at their best.
- Find a restorative exercise like yoga, walking, or swimming, and make it a part of your weekly routine. Avoid high-impact exercise that leaves you drained. Give yourself a break from exercise when you need it, but not for too long – moving the body helps emotional as well as physical well-being.
- Eat well and make nutrition a priority. Plan ahead and keep healthy snacks on hand. When we are rushed and hungry is when we tend to eat poorly.
- Learn how to say 'no' and avoid over-committing in all aspects of your social life and work duties. There are things that we must do and things that we can choose not to do. Learn how to prioritize and think before automatically saying 'yes.' Check in with your emotional well-being. In Chapter

Six, we'll look at the emotional impact of recurrent pregnancy loss and some of the options for getting the help and support you need.
- ❏ Surround yourself with positive, supportive people. Take note of the toxic people in your life and limit or eliminate your exposure to them.

> "Choose people who lift you up."
> – Michelle Obama

- ❏ If you have a partner, make time for your relationship with date nights, alone time, or whatever is best for you as a couple. Remember that your partner is struggling too. Try doing something special occasionally like writing a card or sending flowers – something unexpected on a random day just to let them know you care.
- ❏ Make time in your week just for you – whether this is exercise, lunch with a friend, or quiet time reading a book, schedule something that you want to do just for yourself.
- ❏ Ask yourself, 'What am I going to do for myself today or this week?'

In Summary

Taking steps toward optimizing your health prepares you for a healthy pregnancy and builds habits for a life of better wellness. We all know in general what we need to do to be healthier: eat better, exercise regularly, avoid too much alcohol, limit exposures to toxins – it can be overwhelming, but the key is to move toward better health, step by step. Be cautious of setting goals that are unattainable, like telling yourself you are going to go to the gym every day, because it's easy to give up when you skip a few days. Give yourself a break and be patient with yourself. Do a few things at a time and think about changes toward health, creating lifelong habits that improve your wellness. Make yourself a priority!

Key Points
- Lifestyle modifications that improve your overall health and well-being will improve your chances of a healthy pregnancy.
- Work toward a healthy weight for you in a safe, positive way.
- Eliminate nicotine, tobacco, marijuana, and other drugs.
- Limit or eliminate caffeine.
- Limit or eliminate alcohol.
- Limit exposures to environmental toxins to the best of your ability.
- Make positive choices in nutrition – eat more whole foods and less processed foods as much as you can.
- Make exercise restorative and not strenuous to a point of exhaustion. Exercise is a good thing – get moving!
- Make sleep a priority. Find a bedtime routine that works for you, and stick to it as best you can.
- Self-care is an essential part of your mental and physical well-being, but it does not come naturally to many. You must actively take steps to make yourself a priority.

> **"It's not that some people have will power and some do not. It's that some people are ready to change and some people are not."**
> **– James Gordon**

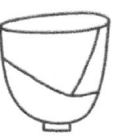

6

Emotional Wellness: The Psychological Impact of Miscarriage

In my medical training, I learned about the diagnosis, treatment, and physical toll of miscarriage, but it's only been through years of caring for patients that I've realized the true emotional toll and psychological impact of miscarriage. I distinctly remember early in my fertility practice calling one of my patients with a positive pregnancy test and hearing a deep sigh followed by heavy silence on the other end of the phone. This was not the reaction of elation and happiness I usually got from my fertility patients who had been struggling to conceive. After a moment, she said, "Thank you, Dr. Shahine. Here we go again." I was stunned, and only after I hung up did it hit me like a ton of bricks – this test was the patient's fifth positive pregnancy test, and for her, this was just the beginning of the limbo, waiting, and anxiety until she knew whether this would be a successful pregnancy or not. For her, this was only a beginning, and she had been down this road before with disappointment at the end. She would be on pins and needles until the next checkup and the one after that and the one after that and would only feel relief once she actually had a baby in her arms.

> The innocent joy of a positive pregnancy test is taken away after miscarriage. We all want the movie storyline with a pregnancy announcement in one scene followed by a baby in arms in the

> next. With miscarriage, the reality that we don't always know the future and that there is no guarantee in pregnancy sinks in. It's part of my work to rebuild confidence and support patients through this difficult time.

Studies have found symptoms of depression and anxiety and signs of post-traumatic stress disorder develop or become worse with miscarriage and recurrent pregnancy loss.[1] Patients report not only a grieving process, with all its stages, but an impact on feelings of guilt and doubts in self-worth that tend to amplify with each loss. Without support and understanding of the common causes of miscarriage, women especially begin to blame themselves for recurrent pregnancy loss (RPL). They blame their bodies, their stress, their diets. Without support and help, this can turn into self-blame and doubts of self-worth.

Men struggle with the psychological impact of miscarriage as well. They can feel angry, depressed, and helpless watching their partner go through miscarriage after miscarriage without knowing how to help or what to do.[2] Every person is different, but I've witnessed in my own practice many men extremely frustrated with a diagnosis of unexplained RPL – they want a problem they can fix, and leaving them with no clear answer is difficult.

Supportive care for patients with RPL is essential. Studies have shown decreased miscarriage rates for women who receive supportive care in the first trimester.[3] The authors of the studies cannot explain exactly why they observe higher live birth rates in couples with supportive care but argue that more contact with medical providers, emotional support through counseling, and comprehensive care should be considered for women with RPL. There is no universal definition of supportive care for patients with RPL; some describe it as counseling and emotional care, close monitoring in the first trimester with serial pregnancy hormone blood tests and ultrasounds, or both.[4] Regardless of how one defines supportive care, all RPL patients are more likely to have signs and symptoms of depression and anxiety and should be offered support and wellness resources as part of their care.

Support and Wellness Resources for Miscarriage

Emotional health is as important as physical health, and every person is unique, with different needs. Below is a list of support and wellness resources that I have found helpful with my patients.

Counseling – One on one or couples counseling can be a wonderful resource for anyone dealing with the emotional struggles and grief surrounding miscarriage. The benefits of a counselor include privacy, individualized care, and an ongoing relationship with someone who can be supportive through future triggers and emotional ups and downs. Patients often decline counseling at first – worried about cost, finding the time for appointments, and other concerns; but those who come back after connecting with the right counselor report feeling a sense of relief and security. Take the time to find the right counselor – someone you connect with who seems empathetic to the roller coaster ride of struggling to complete your family.

Finding a counselor: If you have insurance coverage for counseling, start with your insurer's list to limit the financial burden of care. Ask for references from your healthcare providers, friends, and online. When you call to make an appointment, ask if the counselor has experience with caring for people with infertility, miscarriage, and/or grief. Some counselors and therapists specialize in this area of care. If you do not feel a good connection with one counselor, don't waste your time and money – try someone new.

Support groups – Some people enjoy the camaraderie they find when sharing their own experiences and listening to others share their personal struggles in a support group. Support groups specifically for recurrent pregnancy loss are less common, but support groups for infertility or infant and child loss support groups often welcome patients with RPL.

Finding a support group: Look online, ask your healthcare provider and friends, or call local churches and hospitals. Churches often have support groups that do not require that you be a member of the church and are not always faith-based. If you do not share the same faith as a church with a support group, ask about joining – do not assume you can't. Some hospitals, especially women and children's hospitals, often have support groups available as well. One very helpful national online resource for finding support is the National Infertility Association's website Resolve.org, which has a list of support groups across the United States. Resolve began in the 1970s and has become an excellent resource and advocacy group for infertility and miscarriage.

Mind/Body Program – This is a program designed around the mind/body connection. Its foundation stems from observing biological responses (slowing heart rate, decreased blood pressure) with deep breathing and relaxation techniques at Harvard University in Boston in the early 1980s. Dr. Alice Domar is the pioneer for studying and applying stress reduction techniques to help women with infertility. She runs programs through her Mind/Body Center in Boston, but other therapists and counselors run programs throughout the United States based on her model. The programs usually involve eight to ten-week sessions of weekly meetings in which people learn stress reduction techniques and often share their experiences with others.

Meditation – The practice of meditation has become increasingly popular. Definitions differ, but in general, meditation is the practice of quieting the mind, relaxing, and bringing into focus a goal, a mantra, or a state of being calm. There are many resources for learning how to meditate, including books, online resources, and even apps for your smartphone that walk you through the process. Meditation can be intimidating, but give it a try. Be kind to yourself and try a little each day – it takes practice.

Mindfulness – Mindfulness is a practice of self-awareness and striving to be present in the moment. It is grounded in Buddhist meditation, but it is not strictly meditation. Mindfulness is being present, being aware of your body, your thoughts, your life in a single moment. It is taking time each day to stop, breathe, be aware of sounds, feelings, thoughts. It's a way to quiet the mind and reset, and it can be a useful stress reliever. Mindfulness can be less intimidating than meditation for beginners. There are simple exercises that you can do quickly on your own to try it out. Look for resources online and several books written by Dr. Ellen Langer, social psychologist at Harvard University and 'mother of mindfulness.'

Yoga – Yoga is a group of physical, mental, and spiritual practices that originated in ancient India. Today, yoga is incredibly popular and there are many different types of yoga practice, from slow, stretching, meditative yoga to hot, intense, club-music-pumping yoga. Yoga for fertility has become popular, and many of my patients find yoga improves their physical mobility and decreases their stress. If you have never tried yoga, it can be intimidating at first when the instructor calls out moves and positions you are not familiar with or you are stretching next to someone who can wrap their leg around their head twice. Watch a beginner's video online before your first class, find a studio with beginner's yoga, and forget the other people in the class – we all start somewhere! Don't use the excuse 'I can't do yoga because I'm not flexible' because people do yoga to increase flexibility. Try it!

Self-Care – Self-care is taking good care of *yourself*, and it is an essential part of your overall wellness. In the everyday hustle of family, work, friend, and community commitments, it's easy to put our own needs last. Self-care means putting yourself and your needs first. We reviewed this in detail in Chapter 5, but here's a quick review:

1. Be kind to yourself.
2. Make sleep a priority.
3. Exercise, but give yourself a break from it when you need to.
4. Eat well – plan ahead and make healthy, well-balanced dietary choices.
5. Say 'no' to social engagements and extras at work if possible when you need a break.
6. Surround yourself with positive, supportive people.
7. Nurture your partnership – infertility and miscarriages are extremely difficult on couples. You are in this together – be kind and supportive to each other.
8. Ask yourself, 'What am I going to do for myself today or this week?'

Resistance to Focusing on Mental and Emotional Wellness

I get two strong reactions from patients when I bring up emotional wellness and mental health as a part of healing for RPL. Some patients physically sigh, shoulder melt, and then express a relief that someone is willing to talk about this subject and address their emotions. Other patients quickly shut down the conversation and want to move on to other topics.
I hear:

"I don't have time for that."

"I'm fine – I've got my partner – I don't want to talk to anyone else about this."

"I just want to focus on having a baby – I'll be fine after that."

Well, I humbly disagree. We all need to make time to care for our emotional well-being. We do not know the future, and if the next pregnancy is the baby you're waiting for – fantastic! BUT we don't know that, AND nothing will erase the trauma someone has been through in infertility and miscarriage. Patients with infertility and miscarriage are at higher risk of depression and anxiety in pregnancy and beyond.[5] Infertility and miscarriage significantly increase the risk of post-partum depression. Recovery from infertility and miscarriage can be experienced like PTSD (post-traumatic stress disorder), in which feelings of sadness, anger, and depression may be triggered by memories or life experiences.[6]

> I urge my own patients and anyone dealing with miscarriage to pay attention to the mental and emotional impact of this experience as much as the medical and physical impact. You can develop coping skills and self-care habits now that support you through this current challenge as well as other challenges in the future.

In Summary

Dealing with infertility and recurrent pregnancy loss have been compared to dealing with chronic disease and even cancer. Similar feelings of frustration, isolation, and questions like 'Why me?' surround these conditions, but the reactions from friends and the support provided can be different. As a society, we know what to do when someone gets cancer – we have meals to organize and flowers to send – but people suffering with recurrent pregnancy loss often suffer in silence. Most miscarriages are in the first trimester, before people are physically showing a pregnancy and before they announce it publicly. When miscarriages occur, women so often feel guilty in some way that they don't want to share with friends and family. Even worse, when people have the courage to share, they can find awkward responses from their support network about things they could do differently next time, which just makes them feel even more shame about how their body failed them.

Find the support you need and take care of yourself through this journey!

Key Points
- ❏ Miscarriage and recurrent miscarriage can lead to feelings of depression and sadness.
- ❏ The emotional toll of miscarriage and recurrent miscarriage impacts your relationship with yourself and others.
- ❏ Paying attention to your emotional well-being can be as important as your physical well-being.
- ❏ Find support in counseling, support groups, restorative exercise, books, and online resources.

"Stress is a function not of events, but of our views of those events." – Dr. Ellen Langer, social psychologist at Harvard University and 'mother of mindfulness'

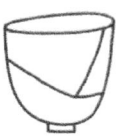

7

The Other Half: What About Men and Miscarriage?

Men contribute half of the genetics of a pregnancy and suffer alongside their partners with loss, but they are so often left out of the research, the care, and sometimes the discussions surrounding miscarriage and RPL. This has been true for all aspects of fertility for decades and plays into society's assumption that reproduction is female-focused and thus, any issues with reproduction must be the woman's fault.

With lack of interest, there is a lack of research, and the role of men's contribution to miscarriage risk is largely unknown. Part of the problem is there is little data and focus on testing to show how men's health and genetics could play a role in miscarriage. Testing for men is largely focused on basic testing like a semen analysis and some genetic screening, but the best way to interpret these tests remains a controversial topic. Fortunately, I've witnessed more research and discussion regarding male contribution to fertility and miscarriage recently than in the past. We still have a lot to learn, but we're heading in the right direction.

In this chapter, we'll review the tests available and treatment options proposed for men with recurrent pregnancy loss (RPL), but keep in mind that this is a very new and under-studied area to date.

Male Partner Testing in RPL

Karyotype for men. This is the only test for men in a couple having recurrent miscarriages recommended by most expert guidelines.[1] It is a blood test screening for a balanced translocation within chromosomes in the male partner of the RPL couple. A balanced translocation is a rare genetic imbalance that does not affect the man's health but puts the couple at a higher than usual miscarriage risk due to a high percentage of sperm carrying genetic imbalances that can lead to miscarriage. (Please refer to Chapter 2 for more details).

Semen analysis. A standard semen analysis evaluates sperm parameters such as count, motility, and morphology (shape of the sperm). This analysis is routinely used as a part of an infertility evaluation for a couple since poor parameters could explain why a couple is not getting pregnant. The role of the semen analysis in an RPL evaluation, however, is controversial. Couples with miscarriages are conceiving, so one can assume there is an adequate amount of functioning sperm to allow conception, but are there parameters in a semen analysis that could explain miscarriage? The American Society of Reproductive Medicine (ASRM) does not recommend a semen analysis for routine evaluation for RPL,[1] but proponents for testing cite some small studies showing poor sperm parameters in couples with otherwise unexplained RPL.[2] Although a semen analysis may reveal some abnormal sperm parameters, current reports do not reveal a direct link between abnormal sperm parameters and increased risk of miscarriage.

Sperm aneuploidy testing. Sperm can be tested for chromosome imbalances (aneuploidy) using fluorescent in situ hybridization (FISH). This test estimates the percentage of sperm with chromosomal abnormalities in a sample. It is assumed that a high percentage of sperm with chromosomal imbalances in a sperm sample would put a couple at a higher risk of miscarriages from chromosomal imbalances. This argument sounds logical, but the downsides to this testing include the following:

1. Not all the sperm can be tested – using information found in a small number of sperm means estimating and assuming what may be present in the whole sample.
2. Not all the chromosomes are tested – usually only five chromosomes (13, 18, 21, X, and Y) are tested, leaving no information on the other 18 chromosomes.

Some studies have shown higher sperm aneuploidy rates in couples with RPL,[3] but ASRM does not recommend routine testing of sperm aneuploidy in couples with RPL.[1]

We've reviewed genetics a lot in this book, and chromosomal imbalance in the embryo is the most common cause of first trimester miscarriage.[1] Some miscarriage genetic testing techniques reveal the parental origin of aneuploidy so that if a chromosomal imbalance is found in a miscarriage, we can identify whether the egg or the sperm made a mistake. A high percentage of chromosomally unbalanced sperm (aneuploidy) would seem to put a couple at risk for miscarriage, but one study looking at parental origin found sperm mistakes in only 7% of miscarriages tested in their sample.[4] This means that in the miscarriages tested, 93% of the time the egg made the genetic mistake leading to an unbalanced embryo and only 7% of the time the sperm made the mistake, and the authors suggest that even if a man in an RPL couple tests for high percentage of aneuploid sperm, that these sperm are weeded out of the selection process early, like at fertilization. If this is true, then testing for percentage of aneuploid sperm in an RPL couple may NOT be very helpful in counseling and guiding treatment.

A logical question from patients who read about this testing is: 'Can we screen the sperm for chromosome imbalances before fertilization and decrease the chance of an embryo having a chromosome abnormality?' This is an excellent question, and I wish we could, but the FISH testing itself destroys the sperm, and for now, there is no technology available to screen for chromosomally normal sperm before fertilization with the egg. We can screen for chromosomal imbalances before pregnancy, but we can only screen embryos (once the egg and sperm have fertilized), and this requires in vitro fertilization (IVF).

> Patients ask about sperm sorting before IUI and IVF, and it would be wonderful to be able to select for only chromosomally normal sperm, but the technology is not available today.

DNA Fragmentation Testing

There are several different tests assessing DNA fragmentation in sperm, and its role in evaluation of male fertility and miscarriage is controversial. Theoretically, the higher the percentage of damaged DNA in sperm, the worse the sperm will function and the higher the risk of miscarriage. Higher percentages of DNA fragmentation have been seen in advanced paternal age, men with varicoceles (dilated veins in the scrotum), and toxic exposures, and some studies show higher DNA fragmentation in men with infertility,[5] but results for men with miscarriages are inconsistent.

Results from any sperm DNA fragmentation testing need to be interpreted carefully before broad generalizations and conclusions can be made about their utility in routine medical practice. The type of testing and the results vary widely from country to country, lab to lab, and test to test.

There are four different sperm DNA fragmentation tests:
1. Sperm chromatin structure assay (SCSA)
2. Terminal deoxynucleotidyl transferase-mediated dUTP nick-end labeling assay (TUNEL)
3. Comet assay

4. Sperm chromatin dispersion (halo) test

Sperm Chromatin Structure Assay (SCSA). In this test, the sperm is mixed with low pH media or heat to 'stress' the sperm, exposing DNA, and dye is added to the sample. The dye will attach to the fragmented DNA and not to intact DNA. A small portion of the sperm (tens of thousands from the millions in the original sample) are put through a flow cytometer machine in which a beam of light shines on the DNA and transmits a wavelength from the light emitted from the samples (one wavelength for fragmented DNA and another for intact DNA). A computer calculates the totals and reports a DNA fragmentation index (DFI). In general, a DFI of less than 15% is reassuring and one greater than 30% is concerning for fertility (and possibly miscarriage) issues. The benefits of this test are that it can screen many sperm (although not all), and it has a standard protocol, which decreases variation between labs.

Terminal Deoxynucleotidyl Transferase-Mediated dUTP Nick-End Labeling (TUNEL) Assay. In this test, 'nicks' or free ends of DNA are detected in the sperm sample by attaching these ends to fluorescently stained nucleotides (like genetic puzzle pieces fitting together). This allows the detection of single and double-stranded damage within the DNA. The cells can be assessed either microscopically or by flow cytometric analysis. A disadvantage of this assay is its many protocols, which make comparison between laboratories difficult.

Comet Assay. This test analyzes approximately 5,000 sperm and can quantify the actual amount of DNA fragmentation per sperm. It measures more types of DNA fragmentation than the other tests (single strand breaks in DNA, double strand breaks in DNA, and sometimes altered base pairs).

Sperm Chromatin Dispersion (Halo) Test. This is a simple, inexpensive kit that measures the intact DNA in sperm. The appeal of this test is the low cost and simplicity, but studies showing its relevance to fertility and miscarriage are lacking.

The degree of efficacy of DNA fragmentation testing for couples with RPL is a controversial topic. Some studies show an association and others do not. One meta-analysis of 12 studies found that combining the findings in these multiple studies showed higher sperm DNA fragmentation in couples with RPL and suggests that this may be a cause for unexplained RPL.[6] However, the studies used different assays for testing and different cut offs for considering what is normal and abnormal. Testing men in RPL couples for DNA fragmentation testing sounds appealing, but it is important to know that:

1. There are several different types of tests, and they are not all equal in reproducibility, accuracy, and relevance.
2. Standard 'normal' and 'abnormal' values have yet to be determined and confirmed.
3. Research linking abnormal DNA fragmentation testing to miscarriage are limited to date.

Research is ongoing for DNA fragmentation, but for now, it is not a part of a routine RPL evaluation.

Epigenetics and Sperm Function

Epigenetics is the study of the impact and influence of the structures around the raw genetic content of DNA that influence which genes are used and how they function. These changes may include methylation (changes in methyl groups) on DNA and chemical alterations in histones surrounding DNA, which either promote or alter the transcription (or reading of) the genetic code laid out on DNA. Investigators state that epigenetics may be the link between environmental impact on sperm resulting in issues with fertility and miscarriage risk.[7] Authors conclude that based on current evidence, we can hypothesize a link between sperm epigenetics, embryo development, and miscarriage, but we need more studies on this theory to make broad conclusions.

If Testing Isn't Perfect, What Can Men Do?

In the field of reproduction, we all want to find a way to evaluate the male partners in an RPL couple. Currently, the only expert-recommended test for men in an RPL couple is a karyotype screening for a balanced translocation. Other potential male-focused testing involves sperm tests that have been designed to evaluate male infertility, including sperm aneuploidy testing, DNA fragmentation, and epigenetics in the sperm. These sperm tests are varied, research into their prediction of miscarriage risk is conflicting, and we are left wondering, what next?

Many men in RPL couples ask for testing and are frustrated when I review what's available. They see their female partner go through a battery of tests of anatomy, hormones, genetics, and immune system, and the men are offered very little. We review all options, and I focus on what they can do to optimize their health and support their partner.

Paternal Risk Factors of Miscarriage

Men, Age, and Miscarriage. The one risk factor in men that may be associated with increased risk of miscarriage is age. The assumption that men are forever fertile while women's fertility is intimately linked to age is not entirely true. Society's assumption that men can have babies at any age (like Mick Jagger at 70!) is simply not true. Fertility decreases with age in men[8] like women, but at a slower rate and less dramatically for most. Some studies show increased risk of miscarriage with increasing paternal age regardless of the age of the female partner.[9] Not all studies agree – some show no difference in miscarriage risk with advanced paternal age.[10] The association of paternal age and miscarriage is controversial and under investigation.

Lifestyle Modifications in Men and Risk of Miscarriage

The lifestyle changes for women we reviewed in Chapter 5 will improve overall health in men as well, so please review that chapter, but this list is more targeted toward men in general:

1. **Maintain an ideal weight** – Obesity has been associated with poor sperm parameters and decreased fertility in men.[11] Obesity impacts all areas of health, so getting to an ideal body weight in a steady, safe manner that you can maintain is an excellent goal.
2. **Nutrition** – Eat more non-processed, fresh, organic, whole food.
3. **Exercise** – Regular cardiovascular and strengthening exercises are good, but there is some evidence to support that high impact, intense, competitive-level training may decrease sperm parameters.[12] Exercise is wonderful, but everything is better in moderation.
4. **Limit toxin exposure** – Think about your food, shampoos, lotions, cologne, and plastics exposure since environmental and reproductive toxins affect men too.[13] See Chapter 5 for specific guidelines.
5. **Quit smoking** – Eliminate smoking and all tobacco use, even smokeless tobacco or vaping.[14]
6. **Limit or eliminate caffeine** – One study showed an increased risk of miscarriage if either partner (woman or man) consumed more than two caffeinated beverages daily.[15]
7. **Limit or eliminate alcohol** – Some research shows that alcohol affects sperm parameters,[16] but there are no universal guidelines for how much is too much. Alcohol is associated with dependency, weight gain, sleep difficulties, and many

health issues. It can be enjoyed occasionally but should not be a part of everyday life and should be used in limited quantities. Patients who drink daily are nervous when I recommend reducing or eliminating alcohol, but when they try it, they usually report back feeling better than ever.

8. **Avoid marijuana** – With the legalization of marijuana in many states, its use will most likely continue to rise. Many patients are not surprised when I recommend quitting smoking or limiting alcohol, but they can be surprised when I recommend limiting or eliminating marijuana. There is a general assumption in society that marijuana is natural and healthy and better for health than alcohol or other drugs. But marijuana has been associated with poor sperm parameters and decreased fertility,[17] and I do not recommend using it while trying to conceive.

9. **Consider a high-quality multivitamin** – Sperm parameters may be improved with a multivitamin, which may help replace some nutrients missing from a man's diet. A balanced, varied diet full of protein, fresh vegetables, and fruit is the best way to meet our nutritional needs, but a multivitamin full of antioxidants may be beneficial. The efficacy of supplements and vitamins for the improvement of sperm function is debated among experts. Studies are weak and results vary.

Emotional Well-Being

The emotional impact of miscarriage and RPL is immense for the couple together, but it's easy for the man's emotional well-being to be ignored. The physical toll of miscarriage is a burden carried by women, but the emotional toll is shared and can be felt in a different way by men.[18] Men often want an answer to the problem or a solution they can focus on and help fix. Miscarriage is gray, not black and white, and the lack of control or direct path to the end goal of a baby can be frustrating for all involved, especially men. Men can often feel guilty watching their female partners go through the physical demands of miscarriage – the changes in their body, the procedures, and the testing. Providers and the field of reproduction tend to focus on women with miscarriage – they are the patients who have the pregnancies – and men can feel like they are watching from the sidelines.

Men are grieving in this process as well, and everyone needs to remember that. Both the men and the women in an RPL couple need to focus on their self-care. Please see Chapter 6 on the emotional impact of miscarriage for a list of resources for emotional support, wellness, and self-care, including counseling, support groups, mindfulness, and more.

In Summary

At this time, there is little research into testing and treatment for men in an RPL couple, but this is starting to change. In the meantime, while we are still investigating men's contribution to miscarriage risk, we cannot ignore their role in the journey for the couple. Men should be a part of the consults for the RPL couple, their questions should be answered, and they can be encouraged to optimize their health both physically and emotionally to improve their overall well-being with the hopes of decreasing miscarriage risk.

Key Points
- ❏ Men are half of the equation in a couple that is having recurrent miscarriages, but research is lacking, and understanding their contribution is limited.
- ❏ Factors in men that may increase risk of miscarriage for a couple include advanced age, obesity, chronic illness,

- environmental toxins, and lifestyle factors, but there is little evidence to support these claims.
- The only test recommended by expert groups for a man in an RPL couple is a blood test for karyotype to evaluate for a balanced translocation (genetic issue found in 3-5% of couples with RPL).
- Other tests like semen analysis, aneuploidy testing in sperm, DNA fragmentation, and epigenetic testing have limited research and limited utility at this time.
- Lifestyle factors that focus on improving a man's overall health and well-being may be beneficial in decreasing miscarriage for the couple.
- The emotional impact of RPL on men is important to remember and address.

"If you're going through hell, keep going."
– Winston Churchill

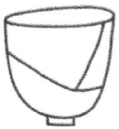

8

Planting the Seeds of Pregnancy: An Integrative Approach to Miscarriage

Recurrent pregnancy loss (RPL) is complex, and Western medicine does not have all the answers. In Western medicine evaluations of RPL, over 50% of patients end up being diagnosed as "unexplained," and these patients are often left wondering what to do next. Many patients ask me about Eastern medicine and acupuncture for all types of medical conditions, and we review options. Eastern and Western medicine have a different approach to care, and together both approaches may help optimize health in preparation for pregnancy.

Western and Eastern medicine approach health in different ways. Western medicine is catastrophic medicine, meaning it is excellent for identifiable problems and crises: you have a broken arm, you see an orthopedic surgeon; you have a serious bacterial infection causing pneumonia, you take an antibiotic. Eastern medicine is preventive medicine and best when used over time. The goal of Eastern medicine is to bring a person into balance and maximize their health using approaches such as nutrition, exercise, and lifestyle modifications.

Western and Eastern medicine providers and treatments are regulated in different ways; there is less regulation and oversight of Eastern care compared to Western care in the US. Physicians undergo rigorous training and testing to become board certified in their field. Prescription medications are regulated by the FDA in the United States and undergo clinical trials, including potential impact to pregnancy. Eastern medicine has the benefit of thousands of years of experience and there is an American Board of Oriental Reproductive Medicine that certifies providers, but not all practitioners are trained in the same way, and there is no FDA regulation or oversight of Chinese herbs, vitamins, or supplements.

I work closely with acupuncturists to provide collaborative, comprehensive care for our mutual patients. Early in my practice at Pacific NW Fertility in Seattle, an acupuncturist named Stephanie Gianarelli, LAc, referred a patient to me. Since that first referral, Stephanie and I have shared many patients and many success stories. We share our different and combined approach to fertility and miscarriage care in our co-authored book, *Planting the Seeds of Pregnancy: An Integrative Approach to Fertility Care*. I appreciate Stephanie's collaborative patient care, friendship, and her help with this chapter on an integrative approach to miscarriage care.

Chapter 8.1: Introduction to Traditional Chinese Medicine

Eastern and Western medicine can work very well together in many areas of medicine, including treatment and prevention of miscarriage. An Eastern approach to care for patients with miscarriages focuses on helping patients find their maximum health and balance before and during pregnancy to decrease the risk of a subsequent miscarriage. In this chapter, we will review the different techniques that Traditional Chinese Medicine (TCM) uses to care for patients who have experienced miscarriage as well as how these patients can incorporate Eastern medicine tools into their everyday life.

TCM is a comprehensive system of medical care that originated over 3,000 years ago and has been evolving ever since. TCM is a holistic form of medicine, focusing more on wellness than disease, correcting subtle imbalances in the body before they evolve into illness. By helping a patient toward a state of optimal health, TCM helps the patient become stronger and readies their body for a healthy pregnancy. TCM can be used to treat disease as well. Through both optimizing health and treating disease, TCM can often help improve the chances of conception and decrease the odds of miscarriage.[1-5]

The four traditional tools or pillars used by TCM to care for patients include acupuncture, Chinese herbal medicine, nutrition, and lifestyle modifications. We will review both the principles behind the use of these traditional TCM pillars in infertility and miscarriage as well as the current research available.

Acupuncture

Acupuncture is one of the most well-known pillars of Chinese medicine. Acupuncturists use the body's energetic framework to balance the flow of Qi (vital energy or life force, pronounced "chee") in the body. If the body's Qi is deficient, in excess, not moving, or scattered, disease often follows. By inserting thin, sterile, single-use needles into acupuncture points on Qi pathways (called meridians), the acupuncturist can help balance the flow of Qi, encourage energy and blood to flow throughout the body, and in turn improve health.

The acupuncture treatment itself lasts approximately 30 minutes and is usually very relaxing. The patient is placed in a comfortable position, either face up or face down, and thin, disposable, sterile needles are placed in acupuncture points on the meridians to help the flow of Qi throughout the body. After approximately 30 minutes, the needles are removed by the acupuncturist, and the patient leaves feeling relaxed and restored.

Acupuncture treatments can include more than just needles to balance Qi. Other methods include moxibustion and cupping. Moxibustion is the burning of herbs (usually mugwort) on or near meridian points to warm the area and alter the flow of energy through a certain point. **Moxibustion** can be direct (burning the herbs on the skin), but most practitioners use indirect moxibustion, in which the herbs are burned near the acupuncture needles or held near the points on the skin to warm the area but not burn the skin directly.

Cupping is another acupuncture treatment that Michael Phelps made famous during the 2016 Olympics in Brazil. Earning record-breaking gold medals, he swam into history with circles of bruises all over his body from cupping. Cupping is an ancient treatment that involves placing cups made of glass or other materials on the skin with suction created either by vacuum or by removing air within the cup with a flame. The suction treatment lasts for 5-15 minutes and leaves the patient with bruises where the cup touched the skin in the shape of the cup. The suction process is meant to bring energy to a certain area and help treat muscle aches and inflammation as well as create balance in the area.

Most acupuncturists recommend treatment approximately once a week, but the frequency and timing in the menstrual cycle are determined by your personal situation. If you are receiving Western fertility treatments in conjunction with acupuncture treatments, be sure to communicate your medications and timing of important treatments like inseminations and embryo transfers to your acupuncturist. Once you are pregnant, your acupuncturist needs to know because they will alter your treatment plan to support your pregnancy.

Acupuncture has been used for thousands of years to treat all aspects of health, including miscarriage, but evidence showing benefits to the standards that we expect with Western medicine treatments are limited. Small studies have shown a benefit to acupuncture in the first trimester in humans,[6,7] and animal studies have shown increased uterine receptivity with acupuncture,[8] but more research is needed.

Chinese Herbal Medicine

A second pillar of TCM used for thousands of years for fertility enhancement and prevention of miscarriage is Chinese herbal medicine. When appropriate, your TCM provider or acupuncturist may recommend a customized herbal medicine treatment, which can come in many forms. Herbal formulas can include:

1. Dried raw herbs, which can be made into a tea by boiling them in water.
2. Granules, which can be dissolved into hot water.
3. Tinctures, which are an alcohol/water blend that has extracted herbal constituents that you take directly.
4. Pills, which can be easily swallowed.

Chinese herbal medicine can be a very powerful way to make the body stronger and replenish what has been lost due to the pressures of modern life, disease, or poor lifestyle choices.

Research also shows that Chinese herbal medicine can enhance fertility and reduce the risk of miscarriage.[9] In one study,[10] Chinese herbal medicine improved pregnancy rates two-fold in a four-month period. And a Cochrane Review of the studies related to Chinese herbal medicine and recurrent pregnancy loss (RPL) showed that, although more quality research needs to be done, Western medicine in conjunction with Chinese herbal medicine may be more effective than Western medicine alone at reducing miscarriage rates.[11] Effects from both acupuncture and Chinese herbal medicine can be enhanced with proper nutrition.

Not all Chinese herbs are the same, and great care must be taken to know what ingredients are in the herbs you are taking, especially when pregnant. Unfortunately, some Chinese herbs have been found to have a high level of heavy metals, which can adversely affect the development of a baby. Please take great care and review options carefully with your doctor before taking any herbs or supplements, especially while trying to conceive or while pregnant.

Nutrition Recommendations

Nutrition is fuel, and what we eat intimately impacts our overall health. Optimizing diet and choosing the right foods and supplements will help bring you into balance and help ready your body to conceive.

Chapter 8.2: Nutrition Recommendations

Include more of these foods in your diet:
- **Plant-based, whole foods** – TCM recommends eating small amounts of hormone-free, organic meat. Sourcing meat carefully whenever possible can decrease exposure to antibiotics, hormones, and endocrine disruptors found in the plastics used in meat processing.
- **Organic, unprocessed whole foods** – Try to make these foods the largest part of your diet. Washing fruits and vegetables (organic or non-organic) will help decrease exposure to pesticides and chemicals used in processing and transporting these foods.
- **Monounsaturated fats** – Like olive oil and avocados. These fats decrease inflammation in the body.
- **High antioxidant-containing food.** Anything dark and naturally colorful, especially beans, greens, and berries, is a

wonderful source of antioxidants, which have anti-inflammatory benefits.
- **Anti-inflammatory foods**:
  - Omega-3-containing foods like cold-water oily fish (herring, salmon, anchovies, and sardines), grass-fed beef, walnuts, flax seeds, pumpkin seeds, olive oil, coconut oil, dark green veggies, cherries, blueberries, turmeric, ginger, garlic, and green tea.
  - Cruciferous veggies (such as broccoli, cabbage, cauliflower, kale, and Brussels sprouts). Make sure that you cook your cruciferous vegetables if you have any type of thyroid issue. Uncooked cruciferous vegetables contain goitrogens that can suppress thyroid function.
- **Bone broth**. Marrow is a very powerful food to make you stronger and build your energy, according to Chinese medicine. Source bone broth carefully, though, since some have tested high for heavy metals like lead.
- **Protein** sources can include lean, organic meats, vegetable-based options, and fish:
  - Non-meat sources of protein can include legumes and nuts. Eggs are an excellent source of protein, but try to find organic, hormone-free, pasture-raised sources.
  - Try to eat more fish that are lower on the food chain, which have lower levels of heavy metals like lead and mercury. Anchovies, salmon, and trout are good choices.

Try to limit these foods:
- **Sugar**. Diets high in sugar lead to insulin highs and lows, and it is tough for our bodies to keep up. Meals with high sugar

content result in spikes in insulin to drive the sugar out of the bloodstream and into our cells for fuel. If we overload on sugar, our bodies cannot keep up, we can become insulin resistant, and our blood sugar levels stay high. High blood sugar levels can be toxic to our cells and lead to vascular injury and long-term health issues like diabetes and its consequences.

❏ **Saturated fats.** These fats provide the building blocks of hormones, constitute a large percentage of cell membranes, enhance the immune system, and provide fat-soluble vitamins like vitamins A, D, E, and K. However, they should be used in moderation. Butter from grass-fed cows is a good source.

❏ **Processed or simple carbohydrates.** Carbohydrates are processed in the same way in our bodies as sugar and lead to the same insulin highs and lows. Eating a balanced diet with some complex carbohydrates is important, but avoid refined or highly processed ones like white bread and white rice. Better carbohydrate choices can include vegetables, whole fruits, legumes, potatoes, and whole grains.

❏ **Trans-fatty acids.** These fats are found in most fried foods, shortening, margarine, and hydrogenated vegetable oil, and they impair the proper functioning of the immune and reproductive systems. Animal studies have shown that high trans-fatty diets result in abnormal sperm morphology, ovulation disruption, and decreased fertility.[12]

❏ **High-mercury-containing fish**, including some tuna, grouper, mackerel, and swordfish. Try to eat more fresh fish in your diet, but if you are eating canned fish, then choose wisely (and limit all canned food due to potential BPA use in containers). Canned albacore (usually called 'canned white tuna') has more mercury than canned skipjack tuna (usually called 'canned light tuna'). Consider canned salmon as an alternative to canned tuna.

Choose beverages that support your health:
- ❏ **Hydrate!** We lose water every day with breathing, perspiration, and other bodily functions, and replenishing this water is essential for staying healthy. We know we need to drink enough water, but how much varies from person to person and depends on factors like activity level, your health, and where you live.
- ❏ **Limit alcohol consumption.** Alcohol has a high sugar content and is tough for our bodies to process. High alcohol consumption is associated with insulin spikes, sleep disturbances, weight gain, and many other health risks. I recommend that patients eliminate alcohol or at least significantly reduce their intake while trying to conceive.
- ❏ **Reduce caffeine intake.** High caffeine intake has been associated with increased miscarriage risk in the first trimester[13] and fetal growth restriction later in pregnancy.[14] From a TCM perspective, coffee negatively affects your overall balance and wellness by expending energy that should be saved. For those patients who love their coffee, I recommend water-pressed decaffeinated coffee. Most coffee is decaffeinated using chemicals like methylene chloride and ethyl acetate (the same chemical that's in your nail polish remover), so look for coffee decaffeinated with water instead of chemicals. Better yet, keep the ritual of a hot drink but switch to caffeine-free tea.

Tips for meeting your nutrition goals:
- ❏ **Plan ahead.** We eat poorly when we are extremely hungry and want something fast. Processed food often contains preservatives and added sugars, and restaurant food tends to

be high in sodium, cooked with trans-fats, and made with non-organic ingredients. Try keeping prepped food like cut-up vegetables and fruits in your fridge. Make one to two meals on the weekends that can last a few days into the week, like soups and veggie/quinoa-based salads that you can take to work with you for lunch or heat up when you get home.
- ❏ **Follow healthy food blogs and websites** that provide ideas for new and delicious meals and snacks.
- ❏ **Share ideas with friends** who are interested in eating better.
- ❏ **Do the best you can**, but don't be too hard on yourself if you eat poorly every once in a while. Remember, "Everything in moderation – even moderation."

Eastern medicine providers will make personal nutrition recommendations for their patients based on their TCM diagnosis. By evaluating a patient physically and learning about their current diet, activity, and stressors in life, the provider will advise their patient to eat more of certain types of foods and less of others to help achieve balance and wellness. Nutrition is an essential pillar of TCM since food is fuel and we are built to get nutrients from food.

Chapter 8.3: Supplement Recommendations

Supplements and Vitamins

Diet is the best way for your body to get the nutrients and vitamins you need to maintain optimal health, and supplements are just that – a way to supplement the essential nutrients and vitamins you may be missing in your daily meals. Food is an ideal way to fuel your body, and supplements or vitamins can enhance intake, but they cannot override an unhealthy diet.

Supplement Recommendations

- ❑ **A high-quality multivitamin.** Supplement your diet with a natural, high-potency multivitamin or prenatal vitamin and mineral complex with iron, folic acid, iodine, and B vitamins.
- ❑ **Fish oil.** Fish oil improves blood flow to the ovaries and uterus,[15] boosts immune function,[16] reduces inflammation, and helps your baby's neural development once you become pregnant.[17] If you are trying to get pregnant, many providers will recommend a daily dosage of 900mg EPA, which helps reduce inflammation, and 600mg DHA, which is needed for brain health in the preconception phase. Note: vegetarian options include flax (flax contains ALA, which converts to EPA and DHA in small quantities) and algae (which provides mostly DHA). Consult with your healthcare provider before taking fish oil if you are taking blood thinners.
- ❑ **Vitamin D.** Vitamin D is essential for utilizing calcium and building strong bones, and it has also been associated with optimizing fertility and reproduction. Vitamin D can be found in many foods like eggs, fish, and fortified milk, and daily sun exposure adds to the body's production of vitamin D as well. I recommend taking a vitamin D3 supplement formulated in oil with a fat-containing meal (fat helps with better vitamin D absorption). Recommendations for daily dose of vitamin D supplements vary from 600IU-2,000IU. Please review options with your provider (including having your vitamin D levels checked) since too much vitamin D can result in side effects like gastrointestinal upset and kidney problems.

Choosing Supplements

Supplements are not regulated like prescription medications in the United States. The Federal Food and Drug Association (FDA) considers herbs, vitamins, and supplements as foods and does not regulate and review these products like they do for prescription medications. There is an assumption that these products are 'safer' than prescription medications because they are more 'natural' and 'plant-based,' but this is not necessarily true. There are many documented instances in which a supplement does not actually contain the ingredients listed on the bottle and even cases of prescription medications being found in supplements sold over the counter without warning labels or prescriptions.

The story of swimmer Jessica Hardy should be a warning for anyone taking supplements. Jessica was banned from competing in the 2008 Olympics because she tested positive for anabolic steroids. She denied doping and after thorough investigation, it was revealed that the diet supplement she took called AdvoCare Arginine Extreme® contained clenbuterol with steroid-like properties.[18] Despite Jessica's due diligence and review of this supplement with her team's nutritionist and contacting the company about safety and ingredients before taking, she missed her chance at competing in the Olympics. What was listed on the bottle was not exactly what she was ingesting, and Jessica paid the consequences.

Please review all vitamins, herbs, and supplements you are taking with your doctor. The National Institutes of Health Office of Dietary Supplements has some key information on dietary supplements on their website. They state that supplements may be used to help ensure you get adequate essential nutrients lacking in your diet, but they cannot claim to diagnose, treat, mitigate, or cure disease. This government agency does not test individual brands and does not recommend any particular brand. They encourage consumers to ask questions of the manufacturer directly, including proof of efficacy, safety of ingredients, quality control in the process, and reports of any adverse outcomes in people taking their product.

So just be aware that claims from a company may not be true and that ingredients listed may not be accurate.

There are independent organizations that test the content, strength, and potential contaminants in supplements. Seals of approval from the following companies do not guarantee efficacy or safety for you, but companies that have these seals are at least willing to have their products tested by an outside quality assurance program:

- ConsumerLab.com's CL Approved Quality Product Seal
- NSF International Dietary Supplement Certification
- US Pharmacopeia (USP) Dietary Supplement Verification Program

Chapter 8.4: Lifestyle Modification Recommendations

- **Avoid endocrine disruptors** such as bisphenol A (BPA) and phthalates (see Chapter 5).
- **Manage stress.** Think about stress as your body's way of preparing you to meet a challenge. Stress can sometimes be impossible to avoid, and miscarriage is inherently stressful. However, research shows that your body's response to stress is not always a bad thing. The destructive part of stress seems to be how we think about it. When we perceive stress as destructive to the body, we increase our risk of disease.[19,20] When we consider stress to be our body's way of preparing us to meet a challenge, stress seems to present less of a health risk.[21] Therefore, working on how we think about stress is more important than trying to avoid the sometimes-unavoidable stresses of life. Be kind to yourself. Try to get enough sleep, try not to work too much, and try to avoid anything too taxing to the immune system. In other

words, give your body every chance to be at its strongest and healthiest so that it can nourish a child.

- ❏ **Unplug.** Disconnect from work, email, social media, and other obligations a little every day. We may feel like we are working hard when we are working many hours straight, but most people find that they can be more productive in a shorter amount of time when they plan for breaks/rest/time off from work.
- ❏ **Clean your teeth.** The bacteria in your mouth can lead to periodontitis, which is inflammation of the tissue around the teeth. The bacteria can then spread to the rest of your body, increase inflammation, and activate the immune system. Studies have shown that bad oral hygiene can increase the amount of time it takes to conceive.[22]
- ❏ **Stop smoking.** Research shows that cigarette smoking is linked to decreased fertility in women[23] and decreased sperm parameters in men.[24,25]
- ❏ **Enjoy exercise.** Low impact activities such as yoga, swimming, walking, and the elliptical trainer are all good exercises for maintaining a pregnancy. Avoid sweating profusely, jarring or abdominal compression exercises, and high-impact activities such as running, particularly after ovulation.

Chapter 8.5: Acupuncture: Tips on What to Expect

Your First Visit With an Eastern Medicine Provider

When people make their first appointment to see an acupuncturist, they are often surprised at the length of both the initial appointment (usually about 90 minutes long) and the intake form (usually five to seven pages long). They often wonder why their acupuncturist cares about their childhood, their likes and dislikes, and their sleep habits, to name just a few of the many questions the acupuncturist will have.

The typical acupuncture intake form covers everything from physical to emotional health history, what you eat, how you spend your time, and the status of your relationships. Each aspect of your life is important to your acupuncturist because each one affects your overall health and wellness.

When you come in for your first time, your visit will begin with an extensive interview covering most aspects of your health and fertility history. Your acupuncturist will then examine your tongue and feel your pulses. The information gathered will be assessed to create a total picture of your state of health.

The acupuncturist will look at your tongue and feel your pulse because visual signs on the tongue and the rhythm and strength of pulses provide insight into the health of the internal organ systems and overall health. This method of diagnosis is subtle and allows the acupuncturist to find emerging patterns of illness rather than just problems that already exist. For example, a swollen tongue indicates fluid retention, a pale tongue indicates deficiency in blood, and a red tongue shows excess heat.

Your acupuncturist will feel your pulse in three separate positions and at three different depths, as each position corresponds to a different organ system. They will look for different qualities in the pulse, such as excess or deficiency. A big pulse, for example, indicates excess heat, while a weak pulse shows deficiency. A pulse that feels like a dolphin cresting under the fingers means an excess in dampness. These are just a few examples in a subtle and comprehensive diagnostic system that has been refined over the millennia.

At the end of your visit to the acupuncturist, you will get a treatment plan customized especially for you. It will cover all aspects of your fertility and overall health. You will be given recommendations on frequency of acupuncture and on appropriate supplements, nutrition, lifestyle choices, and possibly a customized Chinese herbal medicine formula.

In Summary

Miscarriage, and especially recurrent miscarriage, takes a toll on the body and mind of hopeful parents. Eastern medicine can be a powerful addition to your treatment plan, strengthening both mind and body in difficult times and providing support toward your family-building goals. Eastern and Western medicine work very well together. Western medicine is excellent for diagnosing and treating specific causes of miscarriage. Eastern medicine is a more holistic approach, trying to balance your physical and emotional needs to prepare you for a healthy pregnancy. Your Eastern medicine provider can support you before and after conception and guide you to your maximum health. Western and Eastern medicine do not have to be mutually exclusive, and a team approach to care can be a wonderful option for many people.

Key Points
- Western medicine focuses on finding problems and fixing them while Eastern medicine focuses on improving balance and working toward optimal health through treatments and lifestyle modifications.
- Traditional Chinese Medicine includes acupuncture, Chinese herbal medicine, nutrition, and lifestyle modifications to maximize well-being.
- A visit with an acupuncturist will be different from what you expect from visits with a Western health provider – a longer visit with more discussion and education.
- Exercise caution with all treatment options while trying to conceive and especially while pregnant. Some Chinese herbs

have tested high in heavy metals, which can be toxic to a developing baby, so please review all treatment plans with your doctor before starting care.
- ❏ Eastern and Western medicine do not have to be mutually exclusive, and certain aspects of both can come together to benefit patients.

> "Each morning we are born again.
> What we do today is what matters most."
> – Buddha

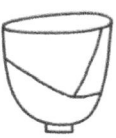

9

Now What? Moving Forward as an Advocate for Your Care

By reading this book and educating yourself about miscarriage and recurrent pregnancy loss (RPL), you are already becoming an advocate for your care. You've learned the medical definitions of miscarriage and RPL, expert recommendations for evaluation and treatment, controversies in care, an Eastern medicine approach to care, and ways to optimize your overall physical and emotional health. Now let's review ways to move forward to find the care that is best for you, what to expect with your visits, and concrete ways to care for yourself that you can start today.

Finding the Right Provider for Your Care

Finding the right provider for evaluation and care for RPL can be challenging. I am often not the first doctor patients have seen for a consult about miscarriages and they often tell me stories of frustration, feeling dismissed, and leaving providers with more questions than answers. This is not uncommon, and it can be related to many factors.

Doctors are people too, and some may feel uncomfortable caring for patients with multiple miscarriages. Unease may result from multiple factors. First, RPL is not common, and many providers do not have a lot of experience caring for these patients – this lack of experience can make providers uncomfortable. Second, most providers do not have thorough or up-to-date training in RPL. Medical training has traditionally been lacking in all areas of reproduction, fertility, and women's health in general. Most research to date has focused on men, and most funding has gone to other areas of health like cardiovascular disease and cancer. Fortunately, this is changing, and we have more knowledge about miscarriage and fertility today than in the past, but unless this is a doctor's area of interest, it's unlikely they will stay up to date with current recommendations for the evaluation and treatment of RPL patients. Finally, many providers are uncomfortable with the lack of certainty or clear answers in RPL. This last one is a tough one for most medical providers. They go to school for years to cure illness and 'fix' people. The thought of doing testing and then having to tell patients that they are unsure why they are losing pregnancies can be scary. Doctors, just like their patients, want to have the answers.

Tips for finding the right provider for you:
1. Some general practitioners and obstetricians have experience with recurrent miscarriage, but many do not. Ask your provider about their experience, what testing and treatment they provide, and when they recommend referring you to a specialist.
2. Reproductive endocrinologists are the specialists for recurrent **first trimester** miscarriages – they are physicians who train in obstetrics and gynecology and then do specialty training in reproductive endocrinology and infertility. Not all reproductive endocrinologists care for patients with recurrent miscarriage, but most will have had the training in their fellowship.
3. Some maternal fetal medicine physicians or perinatologists (a specialty training for high-risk pregnancy after training in obstetrics and gynecology) have a special area of interest in

recurrent miscarriage, but not all. The training for these physicians typically focuses on later pregnancy issues in the second and third trimester, although some will care for women with recurrent first trimester losses.
4. If you are seeing a specialist, ask about their experience, comfort level, and plans for evaluation and treatment.
5. Find someone who will listen to you and answer your questions. A provider with a background in women's health may not have a lot of experience with RPL, but if they are compassionate and willing to learn and help, they still might be a good fit for you.

My miscarriage patients often report frustration when they hear these kinds of statements from providers:

"Miscarriage is common – just try again."

"At least you conceived. That's the first step. It will be fine next time."

"One or two miscarriages can happen, but we do not start testing until you have three losses."

"Just keep trying, there is nothing we can do."

Some of these statements are based on good science, but they could be said in a different way and with more compassion. Most women with multiple miscarriages DO go on to have babies without intervention if they keep trying. The right support team, including your medical provider, can help give you the courage to keep trying. Ideally, you want to find a provider who will say something like:

"Miscarriage is common, but that doesn't mean it's okay or that you're not allowed to ask questions, get an evaluation, and grieve. The majority of the time, the cause has something to do with the embryo – not stress, not that glass of wine you had before you knew you were pregnant, and not that cup of coffee. We should do testing to see if we can find a cause, but even without any testing or intervention, the very next time you conceive, it might be successful. When you are ready to try again, I know a positive pregnancy test is just the beginning, and I'll be with you each step of the way."

What to Expect at Your First Visit: How to Be Prepared

Preparing for your first visit with a provider to discuss RPL can be stressful. You are meeting someone new who may or may not be compassionate, you're going to have to talk about the miscarriages, you're scared they are going to tell you something scary, and so on. Being prepared for what to expect and taking a list of questions with you can decrease your anxiety and make the visit more productive.

Before the Visit
1. **Make sure the office has your relevant medical records.** Do not assume that because the office requested your records or you faxed in a medical release form that the records got to the office on time. Call ahead and double check, and even better, keep a copy of your own medical records that you can bring with you. It's incredible that in this day and age of technology and electronic medical records that medical offices are still printing and faxing records, and you'd be surprised at how often key records are absent from a stack of papers. Keeping track of your own records is a great way to be your own advocate.
2. **Write down your history before you go.** The provider will ask about dates of pregnancies and review what happened with each loss. Consider typing it up and handing the provider this information. Keep a copy for your own

records. It's easy to get confused on dates when relying on memory at a consult (especially when you're nervous). If things are written down beforehand, it will be less stressful and you can spend more time talking about testing and moving forward rather than dwelling on the past (which is important but can also be tough to relive).

3. **Bring a list of your current medications, vitamins, and supplements to review with the provider.** This is good to do because it's easy to forget what you're taking when you're asked on the spot.

4. **If you have a partner, bring them to the visit.** This is helpful in so many ways. First, your partner is having losses too and needs to be a part of the conversation. Second, a lot of information will be covered, and two people listening means a better chance that more will be heard and understood. Third, if you go alone and try to review the visit and what happened with your partner, they will most likely have multiple questions that could have been answered at the visit.

5. **Prepare a list of questions and bring them with you.** If you take some time to write down the questions you want to ask beforehand, you won't get flustered and forget to ask them at your appointment. I've provided a few examples of questions that you may want to ask below. Make sure you bring something to write with to the visit so you can take notes!

At the Visit

Be prepared to review your medical history and obstetric history at the visit. You will likely have blood pressure and other vital signs taken. You may or may not do other testing such as blood work and an ultrasound at that first visit as well.

Hopefully, you'll have prepared a list of questions beforehand to take with you to the visit. Here are some that I would recommend adding to that list:
1. What tests do you recommend?
2. How do I do the testing in terms of scheduling and logistics? Are the tests timed to my menstrual cycle?
3. How will I get the test results – will the office call me? Do I have a patient portal where I can look them up?
4. What treatment will you recommend if the tests do not find a reason for the miscarriages?
5. How can I get my questions answered between visits?
6. What happens if I have another miscarriage? Will you continue to provide care for me? Will you recommend genetic testing on the pregnancy to see if that caused the loss?
7. If you do provide care for me in the first trimester, how long will you follow me into pregnancy? Do you deliver babies too?
8. What kind of support and wellness resources do you have or recommend? Counselors? Mind/body programs? Support groups?

Bring a list of worries with you to the visit as well, and do not be afraid to ask about anything. One of the first questions I ask patients at a visit is, 'What are you worried about?' Patients sometimes seem a little embarrassed when they ask me about some of the concerns listed below, but no worry or concern is silly, and you should just ask!
1. "I'm worried that stress caused the miscarriage."
2. "I started bleeding and had a miscarriage after intercourse with my partner, and I'm worried that sex caused the loss."
3. "I had wine before I knew I was pregnant, and I'm worried I caused the miscarriage."

4. "I didn't stop exercising after the positive pregnancy test, and I'm worried that made me lose the baby."

Remember, no worry or concern is silly – just ask!

After the Visit

Take some time to reflect after the visit. Review your notes and write down what you remember. Do not rely on memory alone – write things down.

That evening, give yourself a break. It takes a lot of courage and energy to have a consult with a provider about the physical and emotional toll of RPL. Have a quiet evening at home or treat yourself to dinner out. Consider a distraction like a funny movie or dinner with friends. Do something for yourself!

Moving Forward

Take time to reflect on all you've learned in this book and move forward toward being your own advocate for care. The longer I care for patients with infertility and RPL, the more humble I get. The field is constantly changing, and we are learning more and more every day. For now, reflect, prepare, and move forward with these reminders and considerations:

- ❏ Find a provider for an evaluation and treatment plan who is right for you.
- ❏ Optimize your physical health:
    - ❏ Optimize your weight in a healthy, positive, sustainable way.
    - ❏ Eat well, limit toxins – remember, everything in moderation (even moderation).
    - ❏ Take a high-quality prenatal vitamin daily and review other supplements with your medical provider.
    - ❏ Exercise regularly with a restorative, energizing routine – not a draining, harsh, exhausting routine.

- ❑ Optimize your emotional health:
    - ❑ Find support.
    - ❑ Be kind to yourself – focus on self-care. This does not mean you ignore others' needs but that you realize that you need to take care of yourself because no one else will, and in the end, you will be a stronger parent, spouse, and friend once you care for yourself.
    - ❑ Nurture your relationship if you have a partner – you are in this together and need to support and be kind to each other.

A Final Word From the Author

I hope you finish this book feeling more knowledgeable and empowered. Miscarriage and recurrent pregnancy loss can leave people feeling isolated, scared, and broken. With education and support, my hope is that you realize that you are *Not Broken* and find the strength to move forward. I sincerely thank you for your interest in this book and hope you found it helpful. Best wishes.

– Lora Shahine, MD, FACOG
Reproductive Endocrinologist and Director of the Center for Recurrent Pregnancy Loss at Pacific NW Fertility in Seattle, WA, and Clinical Faculty at the University of Washington

Glossary of Terms and Acronyms

Abortion: The medical term 'abortion' simply means the premature end of a pregnancy before it can survive independently.

- **Complete Abortion:** A medical term describing a miscarriage that is complete, meaning all pregnancy tissue has been expelled from the uterus, either with or without intervention.
- **Missed Abortion:** A medical term describing a pregnancy that is no longer viable or developing but where the patient has no symptoms of miscarriage like bleeding or cramping.
- **Spontaneous Abortion:** A medical term describing a pregnancy lost without intervention like a dilation and curettage procedure. The term 'abortion' in this case means simply a premature loss of pregnancy and does not include why or how the pregnancy stopped early.
- **Therapeutic Abortion:** A procedure that ends a pregnancy on purpose, either with medication or a procedure like a dilation and curettage (D&C). This term does not indicate why the pregnancy was ended (electively or for a medical reason).
- **Threatened Abortion:** A medical term describing a pregnancy associated with bleeding or cramping but that otherwise seems stable (for instance, if there's bleeding at eight weeks' gestation but the ultrasound is reassuring with an eight-week size fetus with cardiac activity). The term abortion in this case means simply a premature loss of pregnancy and does not include why or how the pregnancy stopped early.

American Congress of Obstetrics and Gynecology (ACOG): The American Congress of Obstetrics and Gynecology was founded in

1951 and is the governing body for obstetricians and gynecologists in the United States.

American Society of Reproductive Medicine (ASRM): The American Society of Reproductive Medicine was founded by a group of fertility specialists in 1944 in Chicago. It is now a multi-disciplinary group with members from many specialties with a focus on reproduction.

Aneuploidy: A chromosomal imbalance in the embryo and the most common cause of first trimester miscarriage.

Anti-Müellerian Hormone (AMH): AMH is produced by granulosa cells in the ovary. Low AMH levels can be associated with diminished ovarian reserve.

Antiphospholipid Syndrome (APS): An autoimmune disorder associated with increased risk of miscarriage. Diagnosis requires clinical as well as laboratory findings.

Asherman's Syndrome: Scar tissue within the uterine cavity that can be associated with difficulty conceiving or carrying a pregnancy to term.

Balanced Translocation: A genetic issue in a patient that can increase risk of miscarriage. This is a balanced exchange of material between two chromosomes that occurs during the conception of the patient and results in an increased risk of miscarriage for that person later in life. It's rare (occuring in <3% of couples with miscarriage) and is diagnosed with a blood test called a karyotype.

Beta Human Chorionic Gonadotropin (BhCG): The pregnancy hormone that is tested in urine or blood to confirm pregnancy.

Biochemical Pregnancy Loss/Miscarriage: A pregnancy that can be detected by positive pregnancy test (blood test or urine test for BhCG) that stops developing before it can be seen on ultrasound.

Blighted Ovum/Empty Gestational Sac: A pregnancy that stops developing around five weeks' gestation. Pregnancies develop in a sequential fashion – gestational sac at five weeks, yolk sac within the gestational sac between five and six weeks, fetus at six weeks next to yolk sac, and fetal cardiac activity between six and seven weeks. If an ultrasound shows an empty gestational sac at six or more weeks' gestation, then the pregnancy has most likely stopped developing and is called an empty gestational sac (the older term is blighted ovum).

Cervix: The bottom portion of the uterus and opening to the uterine cavity.

Clinical Miscarriage: A pregnancy that stops developing after it can be detected on an ultrasound or by a tissue examination (histopathologically under the microscope).

Clinically Recognized Pregnancy: A pregnancy that can be detected on an ultrasound or by a tissue examination (histopathologically under the microscope).

Corpus Luteum: A structure within the ovary that produces progesterone in the luteal phase of the menstrual cycle. The follicle within the ovary turns into a corpus luteum after ovulation.

D&C (Dilation and Curettage): A procedure to empty the uterus that typically involves gentle dilation of the uterine cervix to allow an instrument (curettage) into the uterine cavity to remove contents.

Diminished Ovarian Reserve (DOR): While there is no definition agreed upon by experts, in general, DOR is a state of lowered fertility potential due to either a low number of available eggs, low quality eggs, or both.

Endometrial Biopsy: A procedure in which a tissue sample from the uterine lining is obtained with a small, plastic, straw-like catheter passed through the cervix. The procedure is done in the clinic like a pelvic exam with a speculum to view the cervix (the bottom portion and opening to the uterine cavity). The biopsy is quick but crampy and the patient may choose to take ibuprofen before the procedure.

Euploid: A term meaning a balanced number of chromosomes.

European Society of Human Reproduction and Embryology (ESHRE): The European Society of Human Reproduction and Embryology is the European society for reproductive endocrinologists and others in the field.

Fibroids: Fibroids are basically muscular balls of tissue in the uterine cavity. A more scientific definition is a benign solid tumor made of fibrous tissue of the uterus. Fibroids are common (found in 40-50% of women), and not all fibroids affect fertility or miscarriage risk. Fibroid subtypes include:
- **Submucosal Fibroids**: When all or a portion of the fibroid is located within the uterine cavity.
- **Intramural Fibroids**: Fibroids that are located within the wall of the uterus.
- **Subserosal Fibroids**: Fibroids that are located on the surface of the uterus.

Follicle-Stimulating Hormone (FSH): A gonadotropin hormone produced by the pituitary gland. Its primary action is to recruit and encourage maturation of eggs within the follicles of the ovaries. High FSH levels early in the menstrual cycle (cycle day 3) can be associated with diminished ovarian reserve.

Human Leukocyte Antigen (HLA): HLA is the set of genes that codes for proteins that label our cells as unique. Our immune system uses these protein markers to tell our cells apart from foreign cells.

Hysterosalpingogram (HSG): Hystero (uterus) salpingo (tube) gram (study) is the evaluation of both the uterine cavity and fallopian tubes with contrast dye and fluoroscopy.

Hysteroscopy: A procedure in which a camera is placed through the cervix into the uterus in order to see within the uterine cavity. Some uterine cavity defects like submucosal fibroids, polyps, and uterine adhesions can be treated with this minimally invasive procedure.

In Vitro Fertilization (IVF): The process of conceiving with assisted reproductive technology. In this process, eggs are retrieved after ovarian stimulation with hormones called gonadotropins and are then fertilized outside of the body with sperm in a laboratory. The resulting embryos (fertilized eggs) are then transferred to the uterus for implantation.

Magnetic Resonance Imaging (MRI): MRI is a medical imaging technique using magnetic fields, radio waves, and field gradients to create images of anatomy.

Meiosis: A type of cell division for eggs and sperm in which chromosomes duplicate and then separate so that the parent cell divides into four daughter cells with half of the copies of the chromosomes. There are many stages of meiosis. Oocytes (eggs) are suspended in the meiosis I stage from birth to ovulation. At ovulation, the egg re-enters meiosis and completes the cell division. Mistakes during meiosis can result in eggs with chromosomal imbalances, which can lead to embryos with chromosomal imbalances, which usually results in miscarriage.

Monosomy: Each chromosome should have two copies. Monosomy is the condition in which one copy of the chromosomes is missing. Most embryos with monosomy stop developing early, resulting in miscarriage.

Natural Killer Cells (NKC): NKC are lymphocytes or white blood cells that are important for our immune system and play a key role in successful embryo implantation in the uterus.

Polycystic Ovarian Syndrome (PCOS): A common hormonal imbalance with multiple signs and symptoms that often result in reproductive issues. Expert groups differ in their definition of PCOS, but the most common diagnostic criteria (the Rotterdam criteria) includes irregular menses due to anovulation, high androgen levels apparent either by laboratory findings or clinical findings like extra hair growth or acne, and/or PCOS-appearing ovaries on ultrasound.

Polyps: Overgrowths of the uterine lining found within the uterine cavity; soft tissue similar to skin tags.

Recurrent Pregnancy Loss (RPL): Having multiple miscarriages. The definition of RPL differs based on which academic society you are reading, but as of 2013, ASRM defines RPL as two or more clinical miscarriages.
- ❏ **Primary Recurrent Pregnancy Loss**: Two or more miscarriages with no history of live birth (delivering a baby).
- ❏ **Secondary Recurrent Pregnancy Loss**: Two or more miscarriages with a history of a previous live birth (delivering a baby).

Royal College of Obstetricians and Gynaecologists (RCOG): The Royal College of Obstetricians and Gynaecologists was founded in 1929 in the United Kingdom and is the governing body of obstetricians and gynecologists in Europe.

Saline Infusion Sonogram (SIS): See sonohystogram below.

Sonohystogram: Also known as a saline infusion sonogram or SIS, a sonohystogram is an evaluation of the uterine cavity involving distending the cavity with sterile saline while doing a pelvic ultrasound.

Subclinical Hypothyroidism (SCH): A high TSH associated with normal levels of thyroid hormones. Women with SCH are usually not symptomatic.

Thyroid-Stimulating Hormone (TSH): A hormone released from the pituitary gland that increases the production of thyroid hormones from the thyroid gland. A high TSH level is indicative of an underactive thyroid gland.

Trisomy: Each chromosome should have two copies – the condition in which there is an extra chromosome so that there are three copies present is called trisomy. Most embryos with trisomy stop developing early, resulting in miscarriage.

References

Chapter 1: The Importance of Language: The Words We Use to Define Miscarriage and Why They Matter

1. Practice Committee of American Society of Reproductive Medicine. Definitions of infertility and recurrent pregnancy loss: a committee opinion. Fertil Steril 2013;99(1):63.
2. ACOG. Patient education pamphlet. Available at: http://www.acog.org/Resources-And-Publications/Patient-Education-Pamphlets/Files/Repeated-Miscarriages. Accessed October 26, 2016.
3. Jauniaux E, Farquharson RG, Christiansen OB, Exalto NE (ESHRE). Evidence-based guidelines for the investigation and medical treatment of recurrent miscarriage. Hum Reprod 2006;21(9):2216-22.
4. Kolte AM, Bernardi LA, Christiansen OB, et al. Terminology for pregnancy loss prior to viability: a consensus statement from the ESHRE early pregnancy special interest group. Hum Reprod 2014;30:495-8.
5. Kolte A, van Opperraaj R, Quenby S, et al. Non-visualized pregnancy losses are prognostically important for unexplained recurrent miscarriage. Hum Reprod 2014;29(5):931-7.
6. Zeadna A, Son WY, Moon JH, Dahan MH. A comparison of biochemical pregnancy rates between women who underwent IVF and fertile controls who conceived spontaneously. Hum Reprod 2015;30(4):783-8.
7. Practice Committee of American Society of Reproductive Medicine. Definitions of infertility and recurrent pregnancy loss: a committee opinion. Fertil Steril 2020;113:533-5.
8. Kline J. Conception to Birth: Epidemiology of Prenatal Development (Monographs in Epidemiology and Biostatics, Volume 14). New York, NY: Oxford University Press; 1989.

9. Nybo Anderson AM, Wohlfahrt J, Christens P, Olsen J, Melbye M. Maternal age and fetal loss: population based register linkage study. BMJ 2000;320(7251):1708-12.
10. Du Fosse NA, van der Hoorn MLP, van Lith J. Advanced paternal age is associated with an increased risk of spontaneous miscarriage: a systematic review and meta-analysis. Hum Reprod Upd 2020;26:650-69.
11. Stirrat GM. Recurrent miscarriage. Lancet 1990;336(8716):673-5.
12. Brigham SA, Conlon C, Farquharson RG. A longitudinal study of pregnancy outcome following idiopathic recurrent miscarriage. Hum Reprod 1999;14(11):2868-71.

Chapter 2: Why Me? Evaluation and Treatment of Recurrent Pregnancy Loss

1. Evaluation and treatment for recurrent pregnancy loss: a committee opinion. Fertil Steril 2012;98:1103-11.
2. Jacobs PA, Hassold T. Chromosome abnormalities: origin and etiology in abortions and livebirths. In: Vogel F, Sperling K, eds. Human genetics. Berlin: Spinger-Verlag;1987:233-44.
3. Stephenson MD, Awartani KA, Robinson WP. Cytogenetic analysis of miscarriage from couples with recurrent miscarriage: a case-control study. Hum Reprod 2002;17:446-51.
4. Grimbizis GF, Camus M, Tarlatzis BC, Bontis JN, Devroey P. Clinical implications of uterine malformations and hysteroscopic treatment results. Human Reprod Update 2001;7:161-74.
5. Pritts EA, Parker WH, Olive DL. Fibroids and infertility: an updated systematic review of the evidence. Fertil Steril 2009;91:1215-23.
6. Kolankaya A, Arici A. Myomas and assisted reproductive technologies: when and how to act? Obstet Gynecol Clin North Am. 2006;33:145-52.
7. Varasteh NN, Neuwirth RS, Levin B, Keltz MD. Pregnancy rates after hysteroscopic polypectomy and myomectomy in infertile women. Obstet Gynecol. 1999;94:168-71.

8. Pabuccu R, Atay V, Orhon E, Urman B, Ergun A. Hysteroscopic treatment of intrauterine adhesions is safe and effective in the restoration of normal menstruation and fertility. Fertil Steril 1997;68:1141-3.
9. Buttram VC, Gibbons WE. Mullerian anomalies: a proposed classification. Fertil Steril 1979;32:40-6.
10. Franssen MTM, Korevaar JC, van der Veen F, Leschot NJ, Bossuyt PMM, Goddijn M. Reproductive outcome after chromosomal analysis in couples with two or more miscarriages: BMJ 2006;332:759-63.
11. Empson M, Lassere M, Craig J, Scott J. Prevention of recurrent miscarriage for women with antiphospholipid antibody or lupus anticoagulant. Cochrane Database Syst Rev 2005 Apr 18;(2):CD002859.
12. Laskin CA, Bombardier C, Hannah ME, Mandel FP, Ritchie JW. Prednisone and aspirin in women with autoantibodies and unexplained recurrent pregnancy loss. N Engl J Med 1997;337:148-53.
13. Empson M, Lassere M, Craig J, Scott J. Prevention of recurrent miscarriage for women with antiphospholipid antibody of lupus anticoagulant. Cochrane Database Syst Rev 2005:CD002859.
14. Bahn RS, Burch HB, Cooper DS, et al. Hyperthyroidism and other causes of thyrotoxicosis: management and guidelines from The American Thyroid Association and American Association of Clinical Endocrinologists. Endocr Pract 2011;17:456-520.
15. Alexander EK, Pearce EN, Brent GA, et al. 2017 Guidelines for the American Thyroid Association for the Diagnosis and Management of Thyroid Disease During Pregnancy and the Postpartum. Thyroid 2017;27:315-89.
16. Lazarus J, Brown RS, Daumerie C, et al. European Thyroid Association guidelines for management of subclinical hypothyroidism in pregnancy and in children. Eur Thyroid J 2014;3:76-94.
17. Hirahara F, Andoh N, Sawai K, Hirabuki T, Uemura T, Minaguchi H. Hyperprolactinemic recurrent miscarriage and results of

randomized bromocriptine treatment trials. Fertil Steril 1998;70:246-52.
18. Mills JL, Simpson JL, Driscoll SG, Jocanovic-Peterson L, Van Allen M. Incidence of spontaneous abortion among normal women and insulin-dependent women whose pregnancies were identified within 21 days of conception. N Engl J Med 1988;319:1617-23.
19. Sagle M, Bishop K, Ridley N, et al. Recurrent early miscarriage and polycystic ovaries. BMJ 1988;297;1027-8.
20. Rai R, Backos M, Rushworth F, et al. Polycystic ovaries and recurrent miscarriage – a reappraisal. Hum Reprod 2000;15:612-5.
21. Jakubowicz DJ, Iuorno MJ, Jacubowicz S. Effects of metformin on early pregnancy loss in the polycystic ovary syndrome. J Clin Endocrinol Metab 2002;87:524.
22. Legro RS, Barnhardt HX, Sclaff WD. Clomiphene, metformin, or both for infertility in the polycystic ovary syndrome. N Engl J Med 2007;356:551.
23. Stephenson MD. Frequency of factors associated with habitual abortion in 197 couples. Fertil Steril 1996;66:24-9.
24. Jaslow CR, Carney JL, Kutteh WH. Diagnostic factors identified in 1020 women with two vs. three or more recurrent pregnancy losses. Fertil Steril 2010;93:1234-43.

Chapter 3: When Experts Disagree: Controversies in Care for Recurrent Pregnancy Loss

1. Davenport WB, Kutteh WH. Inherited thrombophilias and adverse pregnancy outcomes: a review of screening patterns and recommendations. Obstet Gynecol Clin N Am 2014;41:133-44.
2. Lockwood C, Wendel G. Practice bulletin no. 124: Inherited thrombophilias in pregnancy. Obstet Gynecol 2011;118:730-40.
3. Evaluation and treatment for recurrent pregnancy loss: a committee opinion. Fertil Steril 2012;98:1103-11.

4. ESHRE Early Pregnancy Guideline Development Group. Guideline of the European Society of Human Reproduction and Embryology: Recurrent Pregnancy Loss. November 2017.
5. Molloy AM. Folate status and neural tube defects. Biofactors 1999;10:291-4.
6. Der Heijer M. Homocysteine lowering by B vitamins and the secondary prevention of deep vein thrombosis and pulmonary embolism: a randomized, placebo-controlled, double blind trial. Blood 2007;109:139-44.
7. Peng F. Single nucleotide polymorphisms in the methylene tetrahydrofolate reductase gene are common in US Caucasian and Hispanic American populations. In J Mol Med. 2001;8:509-11.
8. ACOG guidelines to Nutrition in Pregnancy. Available at: http://www.acog.org/Patients/FAQs/Nutrition-During-Pregnancy#much. Accessed January 1, 2017.
9. Roberge S, Nicolaides K, Demers S, Hyett J, Chaillet N, Bujold E. The role of aspirin dose on the prevention of preeclampsia and fetal growth restriction: systematic review and meta-analysis. Am J Obstet Gynecol 2016;16:30783-9.
10. Velauthar L, Plana MN, Kalidindi M, et al. First-trimester uterine artery doppler and adverse pregnancy outcome: a meta-analysis involving 55,974 women. Ultrasound Obstet Gynecol 2014;43:500-7.
11. de Jong PG, Kaandorp S, Di Nisio M, Goddijn M, Middeldorp S. Aspirin and/or heparin for women with unexplained recurrent miscarriage with or without inherited thrombophilia. Cochrane Database Syst Rev. 2014;4:CD004734.
12. Shaaban O, Abbas AM, Zahran KM, et al. Low-molecular weight heparin for the treatment of unexplained recurrent miscarriage with negative antiphopholipid antibodies: a randomized controlled trial. Clin App Thromb Hemost 2016;23:567-72.
13. Csapo AI, Pulkkinen M. Indispensability of the human corpus luteum in the maintenance of early pregnancy. Luteectomy evidence. Obstet Gynecol Surv 1978;33:69-81.
14. Carbonne B, Dallot E, Haddad B, Ferre F, Cabrol D. Effects of progesterone on prostaglandin E(2)-induced changes in

glycosaminoglycan synthesis by human cervical fibroblasts in culture. Mol Hum Reprod 2000;6:661-4.

15. Csapo AI, Pinto-Dantas CA. The effect of progesterone on the human uterus. Proc Natl Acad Sci U S A 1965;54:1069-76.
16. Druckmann R, Druckmann MA. Progesterone and the immunology of pregnancy. J Steroid Biochem Mol Biol 2005;97:389-96.
17. Murray MJ, Meyer WR, Zaino RJ, Lessey BA, Navotny DB. A critical analysis of the accuracy, reproducibility, and clinical utility of histologic endometrial dating in fertile women. Fertil Steril 2004;81:1333-43.
18. Haas DM, Ramsey PS. Progesterone for preventing miscarriage. Cochrane Database Syst Rev 2013 Oct 31;(10):CD003511.
19. Kumar A, Begum N, Prasad S, et al. Oral dydrogesterone treatment during early pregnancy to prevent recurrent pregnancy loss and its role in modulation of cytokine production: a double-blind, randomized, parallel, placebo-controlled trial. Fertil Steril 2014;102:1357-63.
20. Coomarasamy A, Williams H, Truchanowicz E, et al. A randomized trial of progesterone in women with recurrent miscarriages. N Engl J Med 2015;373:2141-8.
21. Saccone G, Schoen C, Franasiak JM, et al. Supplementation with progestogens in the first trimester of pregnancy to prevent miscarriage in women with unexplained recurrent miscarriage: a systematic review and meta-analysis of randomized, controlled trials. Fertil Steril 2017;107:430-8.
22. Subclinical hypothyroidism in the infertile female population: a guideline. Practice Committee of the American Society of Reproductive Medicine. Fertil Steril 2016;104:545-53.
23. Garber JR, Cobin RH, Gharib H, et al. Clinical practice guidelines for hypothyroidism in adults, cosponsored by the American Association of Clinical Endocrinologists and the American Thyroid Association. Endocr Pract 2012;18:988-1028.
24. Penta M, Lukic A, Conte MP, Chiairini F, Fioriti D. Infectious agents in tissues from spontaneous abortions in the first trimester of pregnancy. New Microbiol 2003;26:329-37.

25. Ralph SG, Rutherford AJ, Wilson JD. Influence of bacterial vaginosis on conception and miscarriage in the first trimester: a cohort study. BMJ 1999;319:220-3.
26. Bouet PE, El Hachem H, Monceau E, Gariepy G, Kadoch IJ, Sylvestre C. Chronic endometritis in women with recurrent pregnancy loss and recurrent implantation failure: prevalence and role of hysteroscopy and immunohistochemistry in diagnosis. Fertil Steril 2016;105:106-10.
27. Chen Y, Fang R, Luo Y, et al. Analysis of the diagnostic value of CD138 for chronic endometritis, the risk factors for the pathogenesis of chronic endometritis and the effect of chronic endometritis on pregnancy: a cohort study. BMC Womens Health 2016;16:60.
28. McQueen DB, Perfetto CO, Hazard FK, Lathi RB. Pregnancy outcomes in women with chronic endometritis and recurrent pregnancy loss. Fertil Steril 2015;104:927-31.
29. McQueen DB, Bernardi LA, Stephenson MD. Chronic endometritis in women with recurrent early pregnancy loss and/or fetal demise. Fertil Steril 2014;101:1026-30.
30. Kwak JYH, Beaman KD, Gilman-Sachs A, Ruiz JE, Schewitz D, Beer AE. Up-regulated expression of CD56+, CD56+/CD16, and CD19+ cells in peripheral blood leukocytes in pregnant women with recurrent pregnancy loss. Am J Reprod Immunol 1995;34:93-9.
31. Katano K, Suzuki S, Ozaki Y, Suzumori N, Kitaori T, Sugiura-Osasawara M. Peripheral natural killer cell activity as a predictor of recurrent pregnancy loss: a large cohort study. Fertil Steril 2013;100:1629-34.
32. Tuckerman E, Laird SM, Prakash A, Li TC. Prognostic value of the measurement of uterine natural killer cells in the endometrium of women with recurrent miscarriage. Hum Reprod 2007;22:2208-13.
33. Michimata T, Ogasawara MS, Tsuda H, Suzumori K, Aoki K, Sasai M. Distributions of endometrial NK cells, B cells, T cells, and Th2/Tc2 cells fail to predict pregnancy outcome following recent abortion. Am J Reprod Immunol 2002;47:196-202.

34. Christiansen, OB, Kolte AM, Larsen EC, Nielsen HS. Immunological Causes of Recurrent Pregnancy Loss. In: Bashiri A, Harlev A, Agarwal A, eds. Recurrent Pregnancy Loss: Evidence-Based Evaluation, Diagnosis, and Treatment. New York: Springer Cham Heidelberg, 2016:75-88.
35. Kruse C, Steffensen R, Varming K, et al. A study of HLA-DR and -DQ alleles in 588 patients and 562 controls confirms that HLA-DRB1*03 is associated with recurrent miscarriage. Hum Reprod 2004;19:1215-21.
36. Nielsen HS, Andersen AM, Kolte AM, et al. A firstborn boy is suggestive of a strong prognostic factor in secondary recurrent miscarriage: a confirmatory study. Fertil Steril 2008;89:907-11.
37. Nielsen HS, Steffensen R, Varming K, et al. Association of HY-restricting HLA class II alleles with pregnancy outcome in patients with recurrent miscarriage subsequent to a firstborn boy. Hum Mol Genet 2009;18:1684-91.
38. Wegman TG, Lin H, Guilbert L, Mosmann TR. Bidirectional cytokine interactions in the maternal-fetal relationship: is successful pregnancy a Th2 phenomenon? Immunol Today 1993;14:353-7.
39. Wang H, Gao H, Chi H, et al. Effect of levothyroxine on miscarriage among women with normal thyroid function and thyroid autoimmunity undergoing in vitro fertilization and embryo transfer. JAMA 2017;318:2190-8.
40. Gomaa MF, Elkholy AG, El-Said MM, et al. Combined oral prednisolone and heparin versus heparin: the effect on peripheral NK cells and clinical outcome in patients with unexplained recurrent miscarriage. A double-blind placebo controlled trial. Arch Gynecol Obstet 2014;290:757-62.
41. Tang AW, Alfirevic Z, Turner MA, et al. A feasibility study of screening women with idiopathic recurrent miscarriage for high uterine natural killer cell density and randomizing to prednisolone or placebo when pregnant. Hum Reprod 2013;28:1743-52.
42. Christianssen OB, Larsen ED, Egerup P, Lunoee L, Egestad L, Mielsen HS. Intravenous immunoglobulin treatment for secondary

recurrent miscarriage: a randomized, double blind, placebo controlled trial. BJOB 2015;122:500-8.
43. Stephenson MD, Kutteh WH, Purkiss S, Librach C, Schultz P, Houlihan E. Intravenous immunoglobulin and idiopathic secondary recurrent miscarriage: a multicentered randomized placebo-controlled trial. Hum Reprod 2010;25:2203-9.
44. Royal College of Obstetricians and Gynaecologists (RCOG). The investigation and treatment of couples with recurrent first-trimester and second-trimester miscarriage. Green-top guideline no. 17. London (UK): RCOG; 2011 Apr.
45. Jauniaux E, Farquharson RG, Christiansen OB, Exalto N. Evidence-based guidelines for the investigation and medical treatment of recurrent miscarriage. Hum Reprod 2006;21:2216-22.
46. Roussev RG, Acacio B, Ng SC, et al. Duration of intralipid's suppressive effect on NK cell's functional activity. Am J Reprod Immunol 2008;60:258-63.
47. Meng L, Lin J, Chen L, et al. Effectiveness and potential mechanisms of intralipid in treating unexplained recurrent spontaneous abortion. Arch Gynecol Obstet 2015;294:29-39.
48. Mowbray JF, Gibbings C, Liddell H, et al. Controlled trial of treatment of recurrent spontaneous abortion by immunisation with paternal cells. Lancet 1985;1:941-3.
49. Wong LF, Porter TF, Scott JR. Immunotherapy for recurrent miscarriage. Cochrane Database Syst Rev 2014;10:CD000112.
50. Porter TF, La Coursiere Y, Scott JR. Immunotherapy for recurrent miscarriage. Cochrane Database Syst Rev 2006;2:CD000112.
51. Scarpellini F, Sbracia M. Use of granulocyte colony-stimulating factor for the treatment of unexplained recurrent miscarriage: a randomized controlled trial. Hum Reprod 2009;24:2703-8.
52. Jacobs PA, Hassold T. Chromosome abnormalities: origin and etiology in abortions and livebirths. In: Vogel F, Sperling K, editors. Human genetics. Berlin: Springer-Verlag; 1987:233-44.
53. Marquard K, Westphal L, Milki A, Lathi R. Etiology of recurrent pregnancy loss in women over the age of 35 year. Fertil Steril 2010;94:1473-7.

54. Katz-Jaffe MG, Surrey ES, Minjarez DA, Gustofson RL, Stevens JM, Schoolcraft WB. Association of abnormal ovarian reserve parameters with a higher incidence of aneuploid blastocysts. Obstet Gynecol 2013;121:71-7.
55. Shahine LK, Marshall L, Lamb JD, Hickok LR. Higher rates of aneuploidy in blastocysts and higher risk of no embryo transfer in recurrent pregnancy loss patients with diminished ovarian reserve undergoing in vitro fertilization. Fertil Steril 2016;106:1124-8.
56. Wald KA, Shahine LS, Lamb J, et al. High incidence of diminished ovarian reserve in young unexplained recurrent pregnancy loss patients. Gynecol Endocrinol 2020;11:1-3.

Chapter 4: Genetics: The Link Between Age, Egg Quality, and Miscarriage

1. Jacobs PA, Hassold T. Chromosome abnormalities: origin and etiology in abortions and livebirths. In: Vogel F, Sperling K, eds. Human genetics. Berlin: Springer-Verlag, 1987:233-44.
2. ASRM Practice Committee Opinion: Testing and interpreting measures of ovarian reserve: a committee opinion. Fertil Steril 2015;103:e9-17.
3. ASRM Practice Committee Opinion: Female age-related fertility decline: a committee opinion. Fertil Steril 2014;101:633-4.
4. Evaluation and treatment for recurrent pregnancy loss: a committee opinion. Fertil Steril 2012;98:1103-11.
5. Demko ZP, Simon AL, McCoy RC, Petrov DA, Rabinowitz M. Effects of maternal age on euploidy rates in a large cohort of embryos analyzed with 24-chromosome single-nucleotide polymorphism-based preimplantation genetic screening. Fertil Steril 2016;105:1307-13.
6. Hassold T, Chiu D. Maternal age specific rates of numerical chromosome abnormalities with special reference to trisomy. Hum Genet 1985;70:11-7.
7. Katz-Jaffe MG, Surrey ES, Minjarez DA, Gustofson RL, Stevens JM, Schoolcraft WB. Association of abnormal ovarian reserve

parameters with a higher incidence of aneuploid blastocysts. Obstet Gynecol 2013;121:71-7.
8. Shahine LK, Marshall L, Lamb JD, Hickok LR. Higher rates of aneuploidy in blastocysts and higher risk of no embryo transfer in recurrent pregnancy loss patients with diminished ovarian reserve undergoing in vitro fertilization. Fertil Steril 2016;106:1124-8.
9. Marquard K, Westphal LM, Milki AA, Lathi RB. Etiology of recurrent pregnancy loss in women over the age of 35 years. Fertil Steril 2010;94:1473-7.
10. Wald KA, Shahine LS, Lamb J, et al. High incidence of diminished ovarian reserve in young unexplained recurrent pregnancy loss patients. Gynecol Endocrinol 2020;11:1-3.
11. Brigham SA, Conlon C, Farquharson RG. A longitudinal study of pregnancy outcome following idiopathic recurrent miscarriage. Hum Reprod 1999;14:2868-71.
12. Hodes-Wertz B, Grifo J, Ghadir S, et al. Idiopathic recurrent miscarriage is caused mostly by aneuploid embryos. Fertil Steril 2012;98:675-80.
13. Murugappan G, Shahine LK, Perfetto CO, Hickok LR, Lathi RB. Intent to treat analysis of in vitro fertilization and preimplantation genetic screening versus expectant management in patients with recurrent pregnancy loss. Hum Reprod 2016;31:1668-74.
14. Murugappan G, Ohno MS, Lathi RB. Cost-effectiveness analysis of preimplantation genetic screening and in vitro fertilization versus expectant management in patients with unexplained recurrent pregnancy loss. Fertil Steril 2015;103:1215-20.
15. Shahine LK. Janet Jackson Pregnant at almost 50 - Wait, What? Available at: https://www.buzzfeed.com/drlorashahine/janet-jackson-pregnant-at-almost-50-wait-what-2c2ty. Accessed January 1, 2017.

Chapter 5: Lifestyle Modifications: Optimize Health and Decrease Miscarriage Risk

1. Blakeway J, David SS. Making Babies: A Proven 3-Month Pregnancy Program for Maximum Fertility. Boston, MA: Little Brown and Company, 2009.
2. Pan Y, Zhang S, Wang Q, et al. Investigating the association between prepregnancy body mass index and adverse pregnancy outcomes: a large cohort study of 536 098 Chinese pregnant women in rural China. BMJ Open 2016;20:6.
3. Boots C, Stephenson MD. Does obesity increase the risk of miscarriage in spontaneous conception: a systematic review. Semin Reprod Med 2011;29:507-13.
4. Lashen H, Fear K, Sturdee DW. Obesity is associated with increased risk of first trimester and recurrent miscarriage: matched case-control study. Hum Reprod 2004;19:1644-6.
5. Lindbohm ML, Sallmen M, Taskinen H. Effects of exposure to environmental tobacco smoke on reproductive health. Scand J Work Environ Health 2002;28:84-6.
6. Venners SA, Wang X, Chen C, et al. Paternal smoking and pregnancy loss: a prospective study using a biomarker of pregnancy. Am J Epidemiol 2004;159:993-1001.
7. Zhang BY, Wei YS, Niu JM, et al. Risk factors for unexplained recurrent spontaneous abortion in a population from Southern China. Int J Gynecol Obstet 2010;108:135-8.
8. Greenwood DC, Alwan N, Boylan S, et al. Caffeine intake during pregnancy, late miscarriage and stillbirth. Eur J Epidemiol 2010;25:275-80.
9. Buck Louis GM, Sapra KJ, Schisterman EF, et al. Lifestyle and pregnancy loss in a contemporary cohort of women recruited before conception: the LIFE Study. Fertil Steril 2016;106:180-8.
10. Stefanidou EM, Caramelliano L, Patriarca A, Menato G. Maternal caffeine consumption and sine causa recurrent miscarriage. Eur J Obstet Gynecol Reprod Biol 2011;158:220-4.
11. Kesmodel U, Wisborg K, Olsen SF, Henriksen TB, Scher NJ. Moderate alcohol intake in pregnancy and the risk of spontaneous abortion. Alcohol 2002;37:435-44.

12. Maconochie N, Doyle P, Prior S, et al. Risk factors for first trimester miscarriage - results from a UK population based case control study. BJOG 2007;114:170-86.
13. Brandes M, Verziden JC, Hamilton CJ, et al. Is the fertility treatment itself a risk factor for early pregnancy loss? Reprod Biomed Online 2011;22:192-9.
14. Conner SN, Bedell V, Lipsey K, Macones GA, Cahill AG, Tuuli MG. Maternal marijuana use and adverse neonatal outcomes: a systematic review and meta-analysis. Obstet Gynecol 2016;128:713-23.
15. Brents LK. Marijuana, the endocannabinoid system and the female reproductive system. Yale J Biol Med 2016;89:175-91.
16. Gundersen TD, Jørgensen N, Andersson AM, et al. Association between use of marijuana and male reproductive hormones and semen quality: a study among 1,215 healthy young men. Am J Epidemiol 2015;182:473-81.
17. Ness RB, Grisso JA, Hirshinger N, Markovic N, Shaw LM, Day NL. Cocaine and tobacco use and the risk of spontaneous abortion. N Engl J Med 1999;340:333-9.
18. Wise LA, Rothman KJ, Mikkelsen EM, Sørensen HT, Riis AH, Hatch EE. A prospective cohort study of physical activity and time to pregnancy. Fertil Steril 2012;97:1136-42.
19. Hegaard HK, Ersbøll AS, Damm P. Exercise in pregnancy: first trimester risks. Clin Obstet Gynecol 2016;59:559-6.
20. Lee EK, Gutcher ST, Douglass AB. Is sleep-disordered breathing associated with miscarriages? An emerging hypothesis. Med Hypotheses 2014;82:481-5.
21. Ratcliffe DA. Decrease in eggshell weight in certain birds of prey. Nature 1967;215:208-10.
22. Longnecker MP, Klebanoff MA, Dunson DB, et al. Maternal serum level of the DDT metabolite DDE in relation to fetal loss in previous pregnancies. Environ Res 2005;97:127-33.
23. Krieg SA, Shahine LK, Lathi RB. Environmental exposure to endocrine-disrupting chemicals and miscarriage. Fertil Steril 2016;106:941-7.

24. Lathi RB, Liebert CA, Brookfield KF, et al. Conjugated bisphenol A in maternal serum in relation to miscarriage risk. Fertil Steril 2014;102:123-8.
25. Minguez-Alarcon L, Gaskins AJ, Chiu YH, et al. Urinary bisphenol A concentrations and association with in vitro fertilization outcomes among women from a fertility clinic. Hum Reprod 2015;30:2120-8.
26. Brieño-Enríquez MA, Robles P, Camats-Tarruella N, et al. Human meiotic progression and recombination are affected by bisphenol A exposure during in vitro human oocyte development. Hum Reprod 2011;26:2807-18.
27. CDC Phthalate Fact sheet. Available at: http://www.cdc.gov/biomonitoring/pdf/Pthalates_FactSheet.pdf. Accessed January 1, 2017.
28. Davis BJ, Maronpot RR, Heindel JJ. Di-(2-ethylhexyl) phthalate suppresses estradiol and ovulation in cycling rats. Toxicol Appl Pharmacol 1994;128:216-23.
29. Hauser R, Gaskins AJ, Souter I, et al. Urinary phthalate metabolite concentrations and reproductive outcomes among women undergoing fertilization: results from the EARTH Study. Environ Health Perspect 2016;124:831-9.
30. Li R, Yu C, Gao R, et al. Effects of DEHP on endometrial receptivity and embryo implantation in pregnant mice. J Hazard Mater 2012;241-242:231-40.
31. Toft G, Jonsson BA, Lindh CH, et al. Association between pregnancy loss and urinary phthalate levels around the time of conception. Environ Health Perspect 2012;120:458-63.

Chapter 6: Emotional Wellness: The Psychological Impact of Miscarriage

1. Farren J, Jalmbrant M, Ameye L, et al. Post-traumatic stress, anxiety and depression following miscarriage or ectopic pregnancy: a prospective cohort study. BMJ Open 2016;6:e011864.

2. Kong GW, Chung TK, Lai BP, Lok IH. Gender comparison of psychological reaction after miscarriage-a 1-year longitudinal study. BJOG 2010;117:1211-9.
3. Liddell HS, Pattison NS, Zanderigo A. Recurrent miscarriage—outcome after supportive care in early pregnancy. Aust N Z J Obstet Gynaecol 1991;31:320-2.
4. Musters AM, Taminiau-Bloem EF, van den Boogaard E, van der Veen F, Goddijn M. Supportive care for women with unexplained recurrent miscarriage: patients' perspectives. Hum Reprod 2011;26:873-7.
5. Farren J, Mitchell-Jones N, Verbakei JY, et al. The psychological impact of early pregnancy loss. Hum Reprod Update 2018;24:731-49.
6. Farren J, Jalmbrant M, Ameye L, et al. Post-traumatic stress, anxiety, and depression following miscarriage or ectopic pregnancy: a prospective cohort study. BMJ Open 2016;6:11.

Chapter 7: The Other Half: What About Men and Miscarriage?

1. Evaluation and treatment for recurrent pregnancy loss: a committee opinion. Fertil Steril 2012;98:1103-11.
2. Zidi-Jrah I, Hajlaoui A, Mougou-Zerelli S, et al. Relationship between sperm aneuploidy, sperm DNA integrity, chromatin packaging, traditional sperm parameters, and recurrent pregnancy loss. Fertil Steril 2016;105:58-64.
3. Ramasamy R, Scovell JM, Kovac JR, Cook PJ, Lamb DJ, Lipshultz LI. Fluorescence in situ hybridization detects increased sperm aneuploidy in men with recurrent pregnancy loss. Fertil Steril. 2015;103:906-9.
4. Robinson WP, Bernasconi F, Lau A, McFadden DE. Frequency of meiotic trisomy depends on involved chromosome and mode of ascertainment. Am J Med Genet 1999;84:34-42.
5. Simon L, Proutski I, Stevenson M, et al. Sperm DNA damage has negative association with live birth rates after IVF. Reprod Biomed Online 2013;26:68-78.

6. Robinson L, Gallos ID, Conner SJ, et al. The effect of sperm DNA fragmentation on miscarriage rates: a systematic review and meta-analysis. Hum Reprod 2012;10:2908-17.
7. Ibrahim Y, Hotaling J. Sperm epigenetics and its impact of male fertility, pregnancy loss, and somatic health of future offsprings. Semin Reprod Med 2018;36:233-9.
8. Sharma R, Agarwal A, Rohra VK, Assidi M, Abu-Elmagd M, Turki RF. Effects of increased paternal age on sperm quality, reproductive outcome, and associated epigenetic risks to offspring. Reprod Biol Endocrinol 2015;19;13:35.
9. de la Rocehbrochard E, Thonneau P. Paternal age and maternal age are risk factors for miscarriage; results of a multicenter European study. Hum Reprod 2002;17:1649-56.
10. Ghuman NK, Mair E, Pearce K, Choudhary M. Does age of sperm donor influence live birth outcome in assisted reproduction? Hum Reprod 2016;31:582-90.
11. Bieniek JM, Kashanian JA, Deibert CM, et al. Influence of increasing body mass index on semen and reproductive hormonal parameters in a multi-institutional cohort of subfertile men. Fertil Steril 2016;106:1070-5.
12. Jóźków P, Rossato M. The impact of intense exercise on semen quality. Am J Mens Health 2017;11:654-62.
13. Estill MS, Krawetz SA. The epigenetic consequences of paternal exposure to environmental contaminants and reproductive toxicants. Curr Environ Health Rep 2016;3:202-13.
14. Sharma R, Haarlev A, Agarwal A, Esteves SC. Cigarette smoking and semen quality: A new meta-analysis examining the effect of the 2010 World Health Organization laboratory methods for the examination of human semen. Eur Urol 2016;70:635-45.
15. Buck Louis GM, Sapra KJ, Schisterman EF, et al. Lifestyle and pregnancy loss in a contemporary cohort of women recruited before conception: the LIFE Study. Fertil Steril 2016;106:180-8.
16. Opuwari CS, Henkel RR. An update on oxidative damage to spermatozoa and oocytes. Biomed Res Int 2016;2016:9540142.

17. du Plessis SS, Agarwal A, Syriac A. Marijuana, phytocannabinoids, the endocannabinoid system, and male fertility. J Assist Reprod Genet. 2015;32:1575-88.
18. Kong GW, Chung TK, Lai BP, Lok IH. Gender comparison of psychological reaction after miscarriage-a 1-year longitudinal study. BJOG 2010;117:1211-9.

Chapter 8: Planting the Seeds of Pregnancy: An Integrative Approach to Miscarriage

1. Rubin LH, Cantor D, Marx BL. Recurrent pregnancy loss and traditional Chinese medicine. Med Acupunct 2013;25:232-7.
2. Magarelli P, Cridennda D, Cohen M. Changes in serum cortisol and prolactin associated with acupuncture during controlled ovarian hyperstimulation in women undergoing in vitro fertilization-embryo transfer treatment. Fertil Steril 2009;92:1870-9.
3. Magarelli P, Cridennda D, Cohen M. Acupuncture and good prognosis IVF patients: synergy. Fertil Steril 2004;82:S80-1.
4. Balk J, Catov J, Horn B, Gecsi K, Wakim A. The relationship between perceived stress, acupuncture, and pregnancy rates among IVF patients: a pilot study. Complement Ther Clin Pract 2010;16:154-7.
5. Piao L, Chen CP, Yeh CC, et al. Chinese herbal medicine for miscarriage affects decidual micro-environment and fetal growth. Placenta 2015;36:559-66.
6. Betts D, Smith CA, Dahlen HG. Does acupuncture have a role in the treatment of threatened miscarriage? Findings from a feasibility randomized trial and semi-structured participant interviews. BMC Pregnancy Childbirth 2016;16:298.
7. Betts D, Smith CA, Hannah DG. Acupuncture as a therapeutic treatment option for threatened miscarriage. BMC Complement Altern Med 2012;12:20.

8. Gui J, Xiong F, Li J, Huang G. Effects of acupuncture on Th1, Th2 cytokines in rats of implantation failure. Evid Based Complement Alternat Med 2012;2012:893023.
9. Yang GY, Luo H, Liao X, Liu JP. Chinese herbal medicine for the treatment of recurrent miscarriage: a systematic review of randomized clinical trials. BMC Complement Altern Med 2013;13:320.
10. Ried K, Stuart K. Efficacy of traditional Chinese herbal medicine in the management of female infertility: a systematic review. Complement Ther Med 2011;19:319-31.
11. Li L, Dou L, Leung PC, Chung TK, Wang CC. Chinese herbal medicines for unexplained recurrent miscarriage. Cochrane Database Syst Rev 2016;1:CD010568.
12. Hanis T, Zidek V, Sachova J, Klir P, Deyl Z. Effects of dietary trans-fatty acids on reproductive performance of Wistar rats. Br J Nutr 1989;61:519-29.
13. Weng X, Odouli R, Li DK. Maternal caffeine consumption during pregnancy and the risk of miscarriage: a prospective cohort study. Am J Obstet Gynecol 2008;198:279.e1-8.
14. Momoi N, Tinney JP, Liu LJ, et al. Modest maternal caffeine exposure affects developing embryonic cardiovascular function and growth. Am J Physiol Heart Circ Physiol 2008;294:H2248-56.
15. Lazzarin N, Vaquero E, Exacoustos C, Bertonotti E, Romanini ME, Arduini D. Low-dose aspirin and omega-3 fatty acids improve uterine artery blood flow velocity in women with recurrent miscarriage due to impaired uterine perfusion. Fertil Steril 2009;92:296-300.
16. Gurzell EA, Teague H, Harris M, Clinthorne J, Shaikh SR, Fenton JI. DHA-enriched fish oil targets B cell lipid microdomains and enhances ex vivo and in vivo B cell function. J Leukoc Biol 2013;93:463-70.
17. McNamara RK, Carlson SE. Role of omega-3 fatty acids in brain development and function: potential implications for the pathogenesis and prevention of psychopathology. Prostaglandins Leukot Essent Fatty Acids 2006;75:329-49.

18. Mathews N. Prohibited contaminants in dietary supplements. Sports Health 2018;10:19-30.
19. Richardson S, Shaffer JA, Falzon L, Krupka D, Davidson KW, Edmondson D. Meta-analysis of perceived stress and its association with incident coronary heart disease. Am J Cardiol 2012;110:1711-6.
20. Nabi H, Kivimäki M, Batty GD, et al. Increased risk of coronary heart disease among individuals reporting adverse impact of stress on their health: the Whitehall II prospective cohort study. Eur Heart J 2013;34:2697-705.
21. Keller A, Litzelman K, Wisk LE, et al. Does the perception that stress affects health matter? The association with health and mortality. Health Psychol 2012;31(5):677-84.
22. Nwhator SO, Opeodu OI, Ayanbadejo PO, et al. Could periodontitis affect time to conception? Ann Med Health Sci Res 2014;4:817-22.
23. Håkonsen LB, Ernst A, Ramlau-Hansen CH. Maternal cigarette smoking during pregnancy and reproductive health in children: a review of epidemiological studies. Asian J Androl 2014;16:39-49.
24. Al-Turki HA. Effect of smoking on reproductive hormones and semen parameters of infertile Saudi Arabians. Urol Ann 2015;7:63-6.
25. Kulikauskas V, Blaustein D, Ablin RJ. Cigarette smoking and its possible effects on sperm. Fertil Steril 198;44:526-8.

About the Author

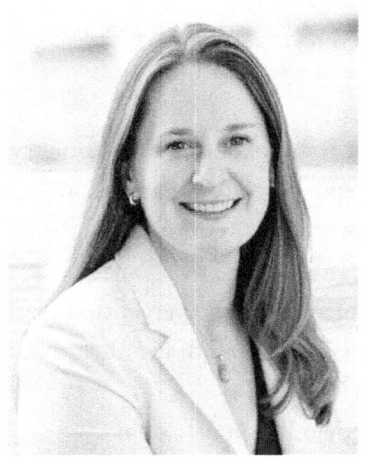

Lora Shahine, MD, FACOG, is a reproductive endocrinologist specializing in infertility and recurrent pregnancy loss at Pacific NW Fertility in Seattle, WA. Originally from North Carolina, Dr. Shahine graduated with a Bachelor of Science in biology from Georgetown University in Washington, DC, and completed her training in medical school at Wake Forest University School of Medicine, residency in obstetrics and gynecology at the University of California at San Francisco, and fellowship in reproductive endocrinology and infertility at Stanford University. She is board certified in both reproductive endocrinology and infertility as well as obstetrics and gynecology.

As clinical faculty at the University of Washington and director of the Center for Recurrent Pregnancy Loss at Pacific NW Fertility, she is committed to providing excellence in patient care, teaching the next generation of women's healthcare providers, and continuing research in the fields of fertility and recurrent miscarriage. She has published over 75 peer-reviewed research projects and is an active member of the American Society of Reproductive Medicine, Pacific Coast Reproductive Society, and Seattle Gynecology Society. She has served on the board of the Babyquest Foundation, a nonprofit organization providing grants to those who need financial assistance with fertility treatment, since 2016. Dr. Shahine is a member of the scientific advisory board of Beautycounter, a B corporation committed to not only creating safer beauty products but increasing awareness and lobbying for stricter guidelines for use of toxins in products.

Dr. Shahine is an accomplished author of many blog posts and articles as well as multiple books. In addition to *Not Broken*, Dr. Shahine co-authored *Planting the Seeds of Pregnancy: An Integrative Approach to Fertility Care* with Stephanie Gianarelli, LAc. She wrote a companion book to *Not Broken* entitled *Not Broken Illustrated: A Gift for Those Who Have Suffered Pregnancy Loss*, an illustrated source of hope and support for anyone who has experienced miscarriage. Most recently, *The Bean Family Sprouts* is her first children's book, reflecting on building resilience and strength through new experiences.

Dr. Shahine is host to the podcast Baby or Bust, which explores the medical and emotional sides to the family building journey one interview at a time.

Dr. Shahine is passionate about changing the conversation surrounding infertility and miscarriage from one of shame and guilt to one of support and empowerment. She lives in Seattle with her family and enjoys travel, skiing, great food, and time spent with friends and family.

More Educational Resources From Dr. Shahine

Website & Blog: www.drlorashahine.com

Host of the Baby or Bust Podcast: www.drlorashahine.com/podcast Learn all about fertility from expert interviews and real life patient experiences.

YouTube: www.drlorashahine.com/youtube

Instagram: www.drlorashahine.com/instagram

TikTok: www.drlorashahine.com/tiktok

Other Books by Dr. Shahine:
Planting the Seeds of Pregnancy: An Integrative Approach to Fertility Care: Exploring Western and Eastern medicine approaches to infertility and miscarriage, co-authored with Stephanie Gianarelli, LAc.

Not Broken Illustrated: A Gift for Those Who Have Suffered Pregnancy Loss: Beautiful illustrations and words of comfort to give to loved ones after miscarriage or stillbirth. Includes resources for emotional support and wellness in recovery.

The Bean Family Sprouts: Dr. Shahine's children's book reflecting on resilience through growth and change, appropriate for any age.

Acknowledgements

First and foremost, I want to thank my patients, the brave, resilient people suffering from miscarriage and facing disappointment but persisting on their journey toward having a baby. Believe me, I've learned as much and often more from you than you have from me.

Thank you to those who have contributed their support and much more to this book – my mentor during my fellowship at Stanford and beyond, Dr. Ruth Lathi, for her forward, Stephanie Gianarelli, LAc, for her chapter on an Eastern approach to care, Lucy Elenbaas for editing, Juli Douglas for her illustrations and cover design, Melinda Torres for her help with design, Judy Simon for her input on nutrition, and Dr. Alice Domar for her input on the emotional impact of miscarriage.

Thank you to my whole team at Pacific NW Fertility (PNWF) for your support of both me and our Center for Recurrent Pregnancy Loss at PNWF.

Thank you to my husband and life coach, Omar. Thank you to my Mom: English teacher, librarian, and my first and favorite editor. And thank you to my Dad, who I watched publish his own book when I was growing up, for inspiring me to be more, do more, and help others (miss you).

Made in the USA
Monee, IL
13 December 2022

21266474R00115